BEE-COME
INDISPENSABLE

John Britt is an international bestselling author with a passion for helping organizations align their strategy with the day-to-day activities and behaviours to reach their goals. He assists companies in effective communication, improved accountability, superior customer service and change capacity. He is co-author, with Ken Blanchard, of *Who Killed Change?*; co-author, with Harry Paul, of *Who Kidnapped Excellence?*; and co-author, with Vaishakhi Bharucha, of *What I Really Meant to Say!* John lives in Louisville, Kentucky, with his wife and multiple pets.

Jan Green is the learning and development officer for Blue & Co. LLC. She is an enthusiastic learning professional dedicated to helping individuals bring their best whether they are just beginning their careers, managing work processes or leading teams to success. Within Blue, Jan has created award-winning development programmes, and most recently Blue received the Learning Elite distinction from the Chief Learning Officer Organization.

BEE-COME
INDISPENSABLE

15 WORKPLACE LESSONS
FROM THE BEES

JOHN BRITT *and*
JAN GREEN

FOREWORD BY HARRY PAUL

RUPA

Published by
Rupa Publications India Pvt. Ltd 2024
7/16, Ansari Road, Daryaganj
New Delhi 110002

P-ISBN: 978-93-5702-731-1
E-ISBN: 978-93-5702-852-3

Second impression 2024

10 9 8 7 6 5 4 3 2

Dedicated to all the working bees who are making the honey and striving to bee-come indispensable in their colony.

Contents

Foreword

Who wants to make themselves indispensable at work? Who wants to be that employee that the boss gives a subtle nod to when the deadline is met, the sale is made, the quota is surpassed or the project is successful? Who wants to be that manager that both the employees and the leadership of the organization know they can count on? Should lean times come again and a team in your organization is sitting around the table deciding what resources they cannot afford to lose, who wants to do everything they can to be on that list?

If you answered yes to any of these questions, then *Bee-come Indispensable* is for you. John Britt and Jan Green have done a masterful job of creating a fun and engaging parable around the working relationships in a bee colony and the behaviours that manifest because of a stressor that has been introduced there. In short, because of 'the hot temperature and the failure of the flower lady to consistently water the garden', the hive is about to experience a honey recession. The parallel between these behaviours and what really occurs in our own organizations is remarkable.

The interactions between Bob Bee (the bee resource director), Dar Bee (a seasoned supervisor) and the worker bees lead us to a better understanding of dysfunctional communication and behaviours. Perhaps, more importantly, it leads to the unveiling of Bob Bee's magnum opus, *Bee*

Attitudes: The Book—a collection of very practical instructions on how we can position ourselves to be successful in our own organizations.

John and I had the opportunity to work together on *Who Kidnapped Excellence?* We both believe that if a reader is going to spend his or her valuable time reading a business or self-help book, we owe it to the reader to help them understand what they should be doing differently today and tomorrow to get a better outcome. *Bee-come Indispensable* absolutely meets that criterion.

Employees and managers, keep this book on your desk or at your bedside. Check yourself against the many recommendations to move toward becoming indispensable.

Leaders, beware! If you read this book, you will want everyone in your organization to have it.

—**Harry Paul**
New York Times Bestselling Author

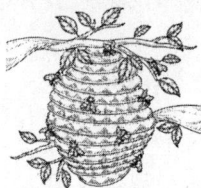

To Bee or Not to Bee?

There was quite a buzz after the Queen Bee left the stage, quite a buzz indeed. As usual, she was succinct. 'The recent weather,' she had begun saying as she hovered behind the podium, 'has not been good for us. The lack of rain, the hot temperature and the failure of the flower lady to consistently water the garden has resulted in a supply chain management problem.'

If she knew the flower lady had been sick, Queen Bee did not acknowledge it. In her mind, one either did their job or did not. And it was this underlying philosophy that had led her to create the slogan for the hive. It was posted everywhere:

To Bee or Not to Bee
That Is the Question We Must Answer Every Day

It was not that she was heartless in regard to the flower lady. Oh, far from it. Most of the worker bees knew that one bee had to lead, to call it like it was, to make the tough decisions, to put the good of the hive ahead of any individual threat or impediment. Queen Bee had been uniquely groomed for this task. And this was all well and good with the hive until her decisions adversely affected the 'Me Bee'.

The 'Me Bee' is what Bob Bee called the worker bees, the frontline bees. They were the ones who did the real day-to-day work to keep the beehive going. Bob Bee was the bee resource director. He had the education and experience and had proven his level headedness time and again. He saw himself as a student of bee nature and knew intrinsically that Queen Bee's speech would stress the organization and cause a myriad of unhealthy behaviours.

After she had indicted the flower lady, she had gone on to say, 'This shortage of pollen and nectar will affect us all. I expect the same level of honey production. We will need to work longer hours and fly further than usual from the hive to survive, to get us through the winter. Are we to bee or not to bee? The answer lies in each and every one of you.'

She had said this with finality and authority. With that, Queen Bee had flown back to her nest.

'Why didn't she talk with me before she made this speech?' Bob Bee said, in almost a whisper.

He was scared out of his wings when a voice behind him said, 'Because she is the Queen Bee.'

Turning around quickly, he let out a sigh of relief when he saw who it was.

'Dar Bee, thank God it's you,' he said.

Dar Bee was one of the line managers in charge of honey production. She and Bob Bee had been friends for years. They trusted one another. Dar Bee saw Bob Bee as one of the corporate bees who really cared about the workers, and Bob Bee saw her as a worker bee willing to speak truth to power. They sometimes disagreed, but they did so in a way that respected the other's position and opinion.

'I smell trouble brewing,' Dar Bee said enticingly.

'Yeah, me too,' Bob Bee replied. 'The last time the colony was stressed by something like this, some of the bees had come out of the woodwork with some unpredictable and almost unbelievable behaviours.'

'I remember,' Dar Bee replied sympathetically. 'But I think this problem is much worse, don't you? I mean a shortage of pollen and nectar—a honey recession?'

'Yes, I am afraid so,' he replied. 'We have so many New Bees. They are going to need some wing holding.'

'That will cut right to the livelihood of the colony. The normal day-to-day operational challenges create enough stress. But this...oh my! Bob Bee, we are going to have to be on our wings for this one.'

'Indeed, we will,' Bob Bee replied. 'Indeed, we will.'

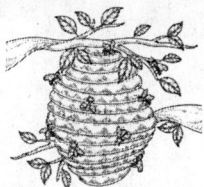

The Bee Attitudes

Bob Bee often thought about when he had started his first job in the hive a long time ago. He had been young and idealistic. He had known exactly what he had wanted. He used to weigh his decisions against his internal sense of right and wrong. And those decisions, those choices, had an impact on how he thought of himself, how he communicated and how he acted. In short, they affected his behaviour. But something had happened over time. That state of readiness, scrutiny and independent choice that he had earlier had somehow faded into his subconscious.

Luckily, Bob Bee had experienced a revelation recently—a wakeup call, if you will. The revelation caused him to understand that some of the behaviours he had adopted were not ones to be proud of. And it became clear to him that day by day, choice by choice, he was the only one who had the power to change himself. And that's exactly what he did. Bob Bee chuckled as he thought about this.

Oh, it's not that I have arrived. I am still learning. Oh yes, I still have so much to learn. But now it is time for me to help some of the other bees. These New Bees, their first few years are critical to wing them with the tools and confidence they need to thrive. And Queen Bee's call for increased productivity will surely exacerbate the behaviours of those who already have a tendency toward negativity. Our worker bees are the backbone of the hive, and they deserve the best opportunity to succeed here!

It did not take long for the negative behaviours to begin. Dar Bee had to write up J. Bee twice.

'What's the issue?' Bob Bee asked Dar Bee. 'How can I help?'

'It's difficult to put a wing on it,' she replied. Dar Bee was lost in thought for a while after. 'Basically, it's his attitude,' she finally said. 'He is so blasted negative and it's rubbing off on the other worker bees.'

'I've read your disciplinary reports,' Bob Bee said. 'It seems you're facing a bit of a challenge in exactly defining the infraction. Is that accurate?'

'That's just it. He just seems to hover right on the edge of a tangible offence but doesn't ever seem to actually go over the line.'

Bob Bee looked at her with the knowing look of an experienced guide.

Dar Bee understood Bob Bee's look and said, 'I know. I know. So why did I write him up you are wondering.' She sighed. 'He's bringing the department down. That's why. I had to do something. If I could get him past this negative attitude, he truly does have a lot of potential.'

'Understood,' Bob Bee replied. 'How about if you and I have a discussion with J. Bee and see if we can sort this out?'

The next day, they met with J. Bee in Conference Room Bee.

'I guess I must be in trouble,' J. Bee said, rolling his eyes. Dar Bee tried to hide her annoyance.

'On the contrary,' Bob Bee replied. 'We've asked you here to give you some choices.'

'Choices?' J. Bee inquired.

Dar Bee cocked her head curiously, but she had known Bob Bee long enough to understand that he had a plan. He said,

'Dar Bee is concerned about you. She asked for my help. It is her impression that you have a way of putting a negative spin on things lately. What are your thoughts about that?'

Dar Bee was a bit surprised at Bob Bee's frankness and also thought that the question he posed was too open-ended. J. Bee looked at her, then at Bob Bee and said, 'Well, all of this overtime and extra flying...what do you expect?'

Bob Bee considered J. Bee's response for a few moments. 'I'll answer your question. I'll tell you exactly what I expect if you don't mind indulging me for a few minutes.'

J. Bee leaned back and put his wings behind his head. 'Why not?' he said.

Bob Bee began his story. 'Not so long ago, I was an angry and insecure bee. I had a general distrust of other bees and felt...well, I felt isolated and like I had to fend for myself to get by. After a while, it was as if the way I responded to others—which was mostly negative, might I add—was just the way I was. It was as if I was genetically engineered to be a negative bee. It was my way of getting what I wanted and needed.'

To her surprise, Dar Bee saw that J. Bee seemed mesmerized by Bob Bee's story and was shaking his head in agreement. Bob Bee continued, 'The circumstances that led me to my epiphany are unimportant, so I won't bore you with the details. But one day, when I was about to unload my ever-present anger on one of my co-workers, I realized I had a choice.'

He looked to see if J. Bee was still with him. He was.

After a few moments of silence, J. Bee leaned forward and asked, 'What do you mean by choice?'

'Well,' said Bob Bee with a smile, 'I realized it was my

choice to be angry or not to be angry. And if I did choose to be angry, I still had a choice of how to respond to it. I realized that the way I responded to circumstances that frustrated me was a choice on my part. It wasn't part of my genetic makeup. It wasn't a latent demon that emerged from the depths of my subconscious. After I made that first choice to not unload on my co-worker, I began to develop a heightened awareness of my emotions. I began to notice that funny little feeling when things seem like they are going wrong...do you know that feeling?'

'I do,' J. Bee said earnestly.

'Well, that is one of my internal indicators to tell the logical side of Me Bee to take control over the emotional side.' Bob Bee paused for a few moments then added, 'But I didn't just stop there though. I mean this awareness of my choices in charged circumstances was a good first step. But with the help of others I was able to understand that for the most part, I could actually choose my attitude on a day-by-day basis. You might ask what the difference is and that would be a good question.'

J. Bee innocently asked, 'What's the difference?'

Dar Bee stifled a smile.

'The difference is that I wake up in the morning and I choose to be positive before any challenging circumstance actually arises. We all have challenging circumstances, right? The difference is that I make a proactive choice in my mindset that keeps me on my wings. So then, when the problem does occur, I have already decided to address it as positively as I can. It makes a difference in my work and my personal relationships.'

J. Bee was awestruck.

'You will ultimately have to make your own choices J. Bee,' Bob Bee continued. 'And the flowers you land on may be different than the flowers I have landed on. But for me, my increased awareness of my responsibilities at work and at home, and my migration to a higher level of self-awareness and self-discipline over time…well, it solidified my relationships and my positions in both settings.'

'Positions?' J. Bee asked, cocking his head.

'Sorry. That was a bit vague. Let me give an example. I believe that because of the things I have just mentioned, my colleagues here can count on me. Queen Bee can count on me. The frontline worker bees can count on me. The important bees in my life can count on me. So, when something like this honey recession comes along, I know that I am trusted and needed. You understand?'

'You have made yourself indispensable,' J. Bee said matter-of-factly.

'Well,' replied Bob Bee, 'I'm not sure that any of us are ultimately indispensable. But I have certainly made myself valuable. Perhaps, we are saying the same thing but from different perspectives.'

'Perhaps,' J. Bee said.

'So, earlier, when you asked me what we expect…we expect you to choose your attitude on a go-forward basis. That doesn't mean you'll turn into a Pollen Anna, of course. That doesn't mean you won't be stressed sometimes. It doesn't mean that you won't get angry now and again. It also doesn't mean that we expect you to turn a blind eye to our issues and challenges here at the hive. On the contrary, we want you to address them. However, we need you to address them in a way that is respectful of every bee here and with an attitude that enlists others to help solve the issues as well. That will happen when you make the philosophical choice to be that kind of bee. When you have done that, you will scrutinize your future choices against those values.'

Bob Bee knew the answer from J. Bee's body language, but he asked the question anyway —'Does any of this strike a chord with you?'

'It does!' J. Bee said immediately. 'It sure does.'

He turned to Dar Bee and said, 'I'm sorry I have caused trouble.'

Dar Bee blushed a little.

Bob Bee stated, 'She came to me because she really didn't want to lose you. Ultimately, she's never lost faith in your potential.'

Dar Bee saw that Bob Bee was looking at J. Bee but past him at the same time. He added, 'J. Bee, if you go down this path, you will begin to have revelations about yourself. It will be exciting. But there will be setbacks. Old habits are hard to break. You cannot let a few setbacks keep you from reaching your potential. You have a great supervisor, me and others who are here to help you succeed. Don't be afraid to come and talk to us if you need help.'

After J. Bee left, Dar Bee said, 'That was pretty amazing. I didn't know you when you were an angry and insecure bee.'

'Actually, you did,' he responded. 'I had made my philosophical choice to be a better Me Bee about a year before we met. I was still working on some issues, but I had learnt some control by then. That is when I started making the list.'

'List? What list?'

'Why, the list of the Bee Attitudes,' Bob Bee said, pulling an old, small leather-bound book from his wingpack.

'Let me see that!' Dar Bee said moving toward him.

Putting the notebook back inside, he said, 'All in good time. All in good time.'

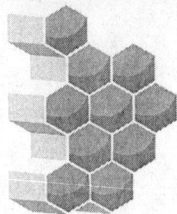

Bee Knowledgeable

Bee Attitude #1

*'Knowledge has to be improved, challenged
and increased constantly, or it vanishes.'*

—PETER DRUCKER

It was Dar Bee who actually facilitated the next hive lesson. Not that she saw it as a lesson. She was just doing her job. She pulled Busy Bee, a young worker bee, aside for a private conversation and began, 'Busy Bee, you are not fanning the nectar long enough.'

Dar Bee could tell that Busy Bee was a little nervous being pulled aside by her supervisor. She was hovering to the left, to the right, up and down at such a pace that she almost became blurry to Dar Bee.

'Take a deep breath,' Dar Bee said. 'I am here to help you.'

Busy Bee slowed a little. 'I don't understand,' she said out of breath. 'The production quota is up. Must do more! Must do it faster!'

'Not at the expense of quality,' Dar Bee replied evenly.

Busy Bee frowned. 'You think I don't care about the quality?' she asked accusingly.

'Now that is not what I said, is it?' Dar Bee replied. 'Let

me explain. When we get the nectar initially, it contains about 80 per cent water. If we do not reduce the water content down to around 15 per cent, the nectar will ferment instead of turning into honey. If it ferments, it is of no use to us. It is primarily you fanning the nectar with your wings that causes the water to evaporate.'

Busy Bee interjected, 'Got it. Learnt that in orientation.'

'What you might have missed in orientation,' Dar Bee persisted, with a bit of an edge, 'is that fanning the nectar faster is not a substitute for fanning the nectar for the required duration.'

She could tell that Busy Bee was thinking. She said, 'I know the increase in the work to produce honey has put a strain on everyone,' she said, in a more conciliatory tone. 'I also know you have good intentions, but you have to understand the fundamental competencies required to get to a quality end-product. We need to look for efficiencies in our work, but there are some processes where we cannot take shortcuts, and this is one of them.'

'Got it,' Busy Bee replied, a bit more relaxed. 'I certainly don't want the honey to spoil. Is there anything else I am missing?'

For the next few minutes, Busy Bee and Dar Bee discussed some of the core processes necessary to keep the honey quality high and what else might be needed to improve production.

Later that day, Dar Bee ran into Bob Bee and told him about her encounter with Busy Bee.

Bob Bee pulled out his notebook, fumbled through the pages and then made a tick mark on it. As he was doing so, he said, 'Ah, a Bee Attitude to check off the list.'

Dar Bee peaked at the notebook and snickered, 'Knowledge

is not an attitude,' she said with a hint of sarcasm. 'Knowledge is…well knowledge is…just that…knowledge.'

Bob Bee returned his notebook to its place and offered Dar Bee a seat.

'No thanks,' she replied. 'I would rather hover.'

Without any sign of resentment at her sarcasm, Bob Bee stated, 'Don't you see Dar Bee. It's the underlying attitude that guides our level of knowledge.'

'Come again?'

'You see, Busy Bee wasn't trying to sabotage the honey. No, it was just the opposite. She was giving it her all without understanding that her current frame of reference, her knowledge of converting the nectar to honey, was flawed,' Bob Bee asserted.

'All correct.'

'And when you approached her with an opportunity to improve her performance, well, she had some choices, didn't she? She could listen or not listen. She could have chosen to be openly defiant, or she could have chosen to be passive-aggressive.'

'All true.'

'Based on what you said, it seems she chose to openly accept your constructive criticism,' Bob Bee said with a smile. 'She opened herself up to your instruction. Not only that, but she also asked what else she needed to know to improve the honey production.'

'She certainly did!'

'That's why I list it as one of the Bee Attitudes,' Bob Bee stated. 'Choosing an attitude that seeks out knowledge so that we can get better at our jobs is a precursor to competency. We need more bees who actively seek the knowledge to improve our production and we need more supervisors like you, Dar Bee, who are willing to have those private conversations to get some of our bees back on track.'

Dar Bee blushed a little. They shook wings and as she was leaving, Dar Bee said, 'I wonder what the next Bee Attitude is.'

Bob Bee went back to his office and opened his notebook to see if there was anything he could add under the 'Bee Knowledgeable' section. Years of experience had taught him two basic lessons. One, that every bee is different. They have different roles, different backgrounds and different perspectives. The second lesson that he had learnt was that because of these differences, not every specific recommendation for improvement was right for every bee. So, over the years, he had added numerous action items that bees could consider improving in each Bee Attitude. To date, this notebook had been his personal resource, but he knew that soon it would be time to share it with the colony.

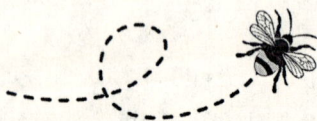

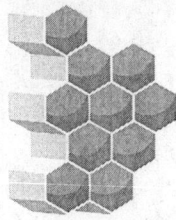

Bee Dependable

Bee Attitude #2

*'Ability is important in our quest for success,
but dependability is critical.'*

—ZIG ZIGLAR

Queen Bee was not happy, not happy at all. Bob Bee had been summoned to her nest, and this was never a good sign.

'How can I help you?' Bob Bee offered deferentially.

Queen Bee was in a state. She was buzzing to and fro. 'I have accountability standards. I go to great lengths to set up expectations,' she droned. 'But does it matter that I go through all that trouble to set up order and structure? Does anyone care that I work day and night, night and day, to ensure the hive thrives? Is it too much to ask for a little accountability?'

Bob Bee and Queen Bee had an unwritten and unspoken agreement that had evolved over time. He was the one bee that she could vent to without fear of it going further. Yes, even the Queen Bee needed an outlet for her frustrations. Bob Bee knew that the rest of the company perceived Queen Bee as austere, perhaps, even aloof. But with him, she occasionally allowed herself to let her guard down. He saw the natural side of her. He considered this state of openness that had evolved between them as a sort of honour. However, he also knew that he had to continually filter the communications between them. He would never intentionally betray her trust.

She continued, 'Accountability, that's right. Accountability. What has happened to their accountability, Bob Bee?'

'How about we start by you telling me exactly what has happened?' Bob Bee said in a low and even tone. 'Who are "they" and what have they done to get you so riled up?'

'I'll tell you exactly who "they" are, Bob Bee. They are the worker bees who are assigned to make sure I have plenty of royal jelly and they, Bob Bee, have failed to provide it two days in a row.'

'Well…' Bob Bee began but was interrupted.

Agitatedly, the Queen Bee said, 'And do you know what happens when I do not get my royal jelly?'

Bob Bee knew, but he also knew better than to talk right now.

'What happens is my ovary development begins to decline. And then what happens?' she asked rhetorically. 'Well, I'll tell you what happens. I stop producing enough eggs to perpetuate the colony. Don't they realize they are putting the whole hive in jeopardy when they fail to do their jobs?'

Bob Bee knew that these actions probably would not put the whole hive in jeopardy. He had seen queen bees come and go, and he knew that if the colony members ever perceived her as dying or weak, they would begin feeding some of the larvae extra royal jelly to develop another queen. However, this he wisely kept to himself. But even through the hyperbole, he saw that she did have a point. After he was sure she was finished talking, he said, 'Why don't I look into it and see if I can remedy the problem. Is that okay with you?'

'Thank you, Bob Bee. Thank you,' she said more calmly. 'You always know what I want. I always know I can count on you.'

A few hours later, Bob Bee met with the worker bees responsible for the royal jelly production. He succinctly and professionally communicated Queen Bee's concern about the inconsistent production of the royal jelly. And he did it without throwing her under the buzz.

'Do you have any idea what it takes to produce royal jelly?' May Bee cast out sarcastically.

'I do not,' Bob Bee replied evenly. 'I leave that to you. You are the experts. But when we do not meet the production standards and Queen Bee calls me to her office, I have to get involved, don't I? There could be very negative consequences to the hive if we do not meet production.'

'You do know we are down several bees?' one of the bees asked.

'No, I didn't know that. How many? Enough to affect production?' he asked.

There was a bit of a buzz among the worker bees. Then, one said, 'Don't know. Hard to tell.'

Bob Bee felt his agenda was about to be hijacked, so he said with authority, 'Let me tell you this in the most straight and civil manner. Queen Bee is not happy. And when Queen Bee is not happy…'

He paused and the worker bees said in tandem, 'No bee is happy.'

They all chuckled a bit and this seemed to lighten the tension.

Bob Bee continued, 'I know you hear me and your supervisors and managers talking about accountability, and you probably think "buzz, buzz, buzz". You think they want to hold me accountable. Translation...big brother bee is looking over my wing to see if he can catch me doing something wrong.'

He felt like he had captured the audience's attention. 'We have, it seems, done a poor job of communicating our expectations. We're not interested in catching you doing something wrong. What we are really looking for are worker bees who are trustworthy and dependable.'

'Can you tell that to my supervisor?' May Bee said cynically.

The crowd was surprised when Bob Bee replied seriously, 'I can, and I will. I will tell it to all your supervisors and managers. Like I said, we have done a poor job of communicating our expectations. We must improve on that.' He scanned the crowd and said, 'We all need to take a long look in the mirror and ask the "to bee or not to bee" question. In this particular case, we should ask how each of us can be more dependable. Can you count on each other? Can management count on you? Can you count on management? Yes, it goes both ways. Will you show up on time? Will you remain focussed to ensure that your part of the work is completed accurately and on time? Will you step up and help your fellow bee when you see them lagging? Will you ask for help when you are having difficulties?'

The worker bees began to hover and buzz.

At this point, Bob Bee had begun to buzz off but turned around suddenly. The buzzing stopped. 'I think it is noteworthy,' Bob Bee said, 'to mention that it is important to ask yourself these same questions about your home, your personal life. Other bees depend on you there as well.'

When all the bees had buzzed off back to work, Bob Bee pulled out his notebook. This time, he added a couple of notes to the 'Bee Dependable' section. He made a mental note to tell Dar Bee about this section the next time he saw her.

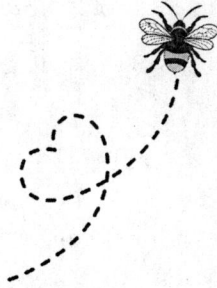

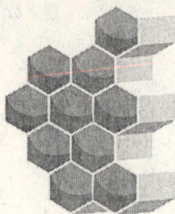

Bee Flexible

Bee Attitude #3

'The measure of intelligence is the ability to change.'

—ALBERT EINSTEIN

'But' Bee was the informal leader of a small group of bees in the hive who always resisted change. Interestingly, he was not what one would call openly resistant nor was he rude as one might suspect of a bee with the label 'resister'. He was called But Bee because the hive could always count on him to begin his sentences with the word 'but' anytime a change was proposed or in play. 'But we've always done it this way' was one of his favourite phrases. Bob Bee was not surprised when he once received information that But Bee was causing a stir.

'You do understand we are trying to salvage the hive?' Bob Bee said, when he met with But Bee.

'But have we truly done an analysis of the current state?' But Bee replied. 'Where are the inventory numbers? You know Queen Bee as well as me and she sometimes shoots from the thorax.'

Bob Bee smiled. 'That's a good question,' he replied.

He thought, *If Queen Bee had consulted me before she made*

her announcement, I would have informed her to include that information in the messaging.

'The inventory supports her position,' he said politely as he turned the inventory report over for But Bee to see.

But Bee perused it. 'But there is no true comparison to last year's inventory. And where's the ratio of production to bee count? Seeing that the production output is down, well that is all well and good but it's really a matter of the honey to bee ratio, isn't it? If I am not incorrect, we have less bees now?'

Bob Bee turned the report to the next page which had the heading 'Honey to Bee Ratio'. He allowed But Bee time to digest the content. After a few moments, But Bee said, 'Okay, I see the ratio of honey to bees has actually improved, but where's the evidence to support Queen Bee's plan? Does she not understand that flying further and working longer hours expends more energy and will require increased resource consumption to sustain such a pace?'

Bob Bee again turned the page for But Bee. The next page was titled 'Honey/Energy Diminishing Return Breakpoint'. But Bee looked over the analysis which asserted that the point of diminishing return was well outside the scope of what Queen Bee was asking of her hive. Looking back up at Bob Bee, he said, 'But this is not the way we have done things around here. There is no assurance her plan will work.'

Bob Bee knew that he had reached the heart of the matter now. The phrase 'that's not the way we have done things around here' was representative of trying to keep a grip on the status quo when something new was on the horizon. After all, so far the status quo represented success and change only offered ambiguity and just a mere chance of success. He began his conversation in earnest with But Bee.

An hour later, as Dar Bee was coming to Bob Bee's office she saw him and But Bee smiling and winging each other on the back as But Bee was leaving.

'So, how did it go?' Dar Bee asked with interest when she was alone with Bob Bee. He had informed her the previous day that he was going to have a talk with But Bee.

'Very well. Very well, indeed,' Bob Bee responded enthusiastically.

'Well, But Bee was certainly smiling when he left.'

But Bee was also known for always having an inscrutable look on his face. Many even said it was a sour look that was representative of his pessimistic outlook. 'How did you do it?' Dar Bee asked.

Bob Bee offered Dar Bee a ration of honey. She gladly took it. 'Well,' he began, 'as you are well aware, But Bee has been labelled a resister.' Dar Bee nodded in agreement. She was then surprised when he said, 'That's not how I see But Bee.' He paused, then said, 'I believe that what we often label as resistance is actually more in the category of reluctance.'

'Interesting,' Dar Bee said and then tasted her honey.

'Some of the bees have legitimate questions and concerns when there is a change like this. If we don't give them a platform to ask and have those questions and concerns addressed, quite often bees with personalities like But Bee—you know…assertive, not scared to give their opinion to anyone—well, they become the de facto voice for these bees.'

Bob Bee stared past Dar Bee for several moments. Then, he said, 'You see, we view bees like But Bee as "against management". Don't get me wrong, there may be a few who are just that. We must be careful, however, because many of these bees are often committed bees who just want to know that their energy and work is going to make a difference.'

'You think But Bee was just reluctant then?'

'Anxious and reluctant,' replied Bob Bee. 'Those unanswered questions and concerns can lead to a high level of anxiety.' Bob Bee slipped into teaching mode, and said, 'A big change is a two-way street, you see. There are the bees that are leading and managing the change and then there are the followers. The leaders and managers provide the vision for the change, the guidance and the resources. The followers, in our case the worker bees, are the ones executing the changes.'

Dar Bee nodded in agreement.

'When you were on the frontlines, Dar Bee, and a big change came along, what went through your head? What questions and concerns did you have?'

Dar Bee wrinkled her head in thought and then began to spout off a list: 'What is the change?; Why are we changing now?; Is something not working?; How will it affect me?'

She looked up at Bob Bee.

'There are certainly more questions but those are the big four,' he said. 'And the last one you mentioned, well, most bees have their antennae pointed toward the same radio station: WIFMB.'

Dar Bee looked at him inquisitively. Bob Bee smiled wryly and said, 'What's in it for Me Bee?'

Dar Bee smiled and said, 'I think that's just bee nature, don't you?'

'All bees have these questions when a big change comes along,' Bob Bee said nodding his head in agreement. 'Some, like But Bee, will ask the questions. But others, who are not so outspoken, might not. We have the responsibility to address these questions and concerns whether they are asked out loud or not.'

'And the worker bees' responsibilities?'

'Well,' began Bob Bee, 'you know these bees have different personalities. But in general, I would advise them to ask the questions. State the concerns. And to do so in a manner that is respectful and professional.'

'Anything else?' Dar Bee asked.

Bob Bee considered. 'Yes,' he finally said. 'Whether it is a colony-wide, significant change or a smaller departmental change, I would encourage every bee to adopt an attitude of flexibility. We must move away from that adage "that's the way we've always done it". Particularly in stressful or challenging times, the bees who can adopt and adapt, well, those bees are extremely valuable.'

'I suppose flexibility is one of your sacred Bee Attitudes,' Dar Bee teased.

Bob Bee pulled out his list, made a check mark on it and smiled as he kept it back. Later that evening, he pulled it out again to see if he needed to add anything to it.

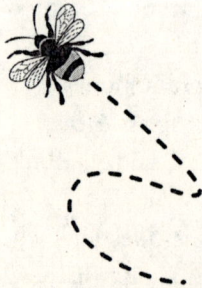

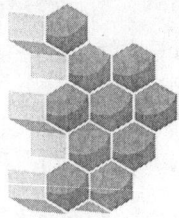

Bee Innovative

Bee Attitude #4

'I am looking for a lot of men who have an infinite capacity to not know what can't be done.'

—HENRY FORD

One day, Dar Bee invited Bob Bee to meet her at one of the hive departments. He could see that she was all excited about something.

'You are probably wondering why I brought you here,' Dar Bee said enthusiastically. Without allowing him time to answer, she said, 'Well, do you remember when Queen Bee said we will need to work longer hours and fly further than usual in order to survive when she gave her speech?'

'I do.'

'And do you remember the sense of dread we felt when she said this?'

'I do.'

Dar Bee pulled out her notebook and excitedly stated, 'Look at these.'

Bob Bee was familiar with the reports. Slowly, he turned the pages. After a few minutes, he looked up at Dar Bee and summarily stated, 'Production for this department is up 6 per cent and no overtime.'

'Exactly!' Dar Bee exclaimed.

Bob Bee put forth the obvious question. 'How are they doing it?'

'Why don't we hear the answer directly from the bee who led the way on this?'

Dar Bee left and returned in a few moments with another bee.

'Rig Bee, eh?' Bob Bee said, shaking her wing, 'Dar Bee tells me that you have apparently worked some production magic.'

'Oh no, not magic,' Rig Bee replied. Bob Bee sensed true humility in her voice. 'We took Queen Bee's speech as a challenge.'

'A challenge?' inquired Bob Bee.

'Yes, but not in a negative way,' Rig Bee replied. 'None of us really care for working overtime, so we got together to discuss how we might be able to meet the same production quotas without overtime.'

'You did this on your own?' Bob Bee asked respectfully.

Rig Bee hovered to her left and then to her right and looked over each wing suspiciously. 'To be honest,' she said in a hushed tone, 'We all knew we had opportunities to improve production without this challenge from Queen Bee as well. It just made a lot of sense for us to try to close the gaps on these opportunities before we started working longer hours.'

Nodding at Dar Bee's reports, Bob Bee offered, 'It seems like it is paying off. Can you give me some examples of what you did to get these types of results?'

'We started with redundant work,' Rig Bee began. 'We all knew there was a nominal amount of redundancy in our approach to our work but until we openly communicated our processes, we had no idea how high the redundancy level was. We redefined the processes to reduce the redundancy and that freed up some of the bees' time to accomplish other, more productive, functions.'

'Makes a lot of sense,' Dar Bee interjected.

'Then we focussed on defects,' Rig Bee continued.

'Defects?' asked Bob Bee.

'You know. Work that has errors in it or work that perhaps lacks something of value.'

'I get the errors part, but I am not sure I understand what you mean when you say "lacks something of value",' Bob Bee said with great interest.

'Good question,' Rig Bee replied. 'We started at the end. What I mean by that is we began with the objective of at least maintaining the previous level of production and we worked backwards. We examined every step of our production process and tagged those activities that did not make a difference in meeting the objective. If they did not make a difference, then they were not adding value. We simply redesigned our processes and deleted many of those activities. Again, this freed up some time for our worker bees to do something that did add value.'

'Wow!' Bob Bee exclaimed. 'Like a modified root-cause analysis of sorts.'

'Exactly,' Rig Bee answered. After a few more minor comments about what her team did to improve production in the face of the challenge, Rig Bee declared that she must get back to work.

After she left, Dar Bee eyed Bob Bee knowingly and inquired, 'One of your Bee Attitudes, I suppose?'

'Absolutely!' replied Bob Bee. 'We want our bees to be innovative. We don't want a bunch of automatons working here. We want bees who can use their brain and their ingenuity.'

'This from the bee who thrives on policy and procedure,' Dar Bee said with light sarcasm.

'Oh, don't get me wrong,' he replied. 'Every hive needs structure, a sense of order. There is no doubt about that. Order breeds predictability and predictability, in turn, fosters security. We owe that to our workers.'

'Well said,' Dar Bee put in.

'But we must also give our bees some space for their ideas, thoughts and potential solutions. If I have learnt anything in my years here, it is that if we can create a culture that gives our frontline bees a voice in how they can do their work more effectively, we will not be let down. That is our job.'

'Then we need more bees like Rig Bee to step up!' Dar Bee declared. Bob Bee patted his Bee Attitude notebook and said, 'I will make some additions to this later tonight.'

'When are you going to let me see that thing?' Dar Bee asked.

'Soon!' Bob Bee replied. 'Very soon.'

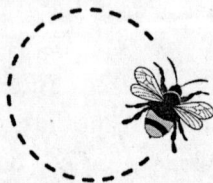

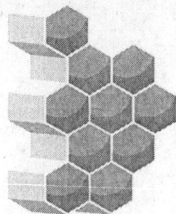

Bee Authentic

Bee Attitude #5

'*We are constantly invited to be what we are.*'

—HENRY DAVID THOREAU

In word and deed, Bogus Bee flew under the radar. He was the first to offer a solution when a problem was identified in a meeting, but he was the last to volunteer to do the real work that flowed from the suggestion. And somehow, he was the first bee the Boss noticed when she came into the hive department. 'Busy as a bee!' she would say with a chuckle. And yet, he was the last bee to arrive at work and the first bee to leave at the nearing of the shift's end.

One day, Dar Bee was trying to describe Bogus Bee's elusive behaviour to Bob Bee. She finished her rambling monologue lamely, saying, 'I just think he has a poor work ethic.'

'Maybe,' Bob Bee offered.

'Or?' Dar Bee asked.

'Or maybe these behaviours you have described are a manifestation of a more latent issue?'

'Well, when did you get your psychology licence?' Dar Bee inquired jokingly.

Bob Bee blushed a little. 'Oh no, no,' he replied. 'I am just a humble student of bee behaviour. I'm just wondering if he has issues with authenticity.'

'Authenticity?'

'Does he joke around a lot?'

'Yes.'

'Does he avoid meaningful issues?'

'Yes.'

'Does he exaggerate?'

'Yes, sometimes.'

'Do you ever have the feeling he is misrepresenting data or information?'

Dar Bee hesitated, and Bob Bee read her body language and began to soothe her, saying, 'I don't mean...'

Dar Bee interrupted him saying, 'Sorry, but I think you have hit the stinger on the head. I am always sceptical of what he has to say.' She paused and then added, 'I don't even think he is consciously being dishonest.' She then corrected herself immediately, saying, 'Dishonest is much too strong a word.'

'I am getting the picture,' Bob Bee interjected. 'It is quite possible that a cognitive dissonance exists between the behaviour Bogus Bee thinks we want from him and his true nature.'

'My, my doctor Bob Bee,' Dar Bee said with a wing salute. 'D-i-s-s-o-n-a-n-c-e,' she spelled out and while bowing, added, 'I must ask you to reduce your high-minded vernacular down into laybee's terms please.'

Bob Bee gestured dismissively at her jokes. 'All I am saying is that he may believe that what the hive needs from him doesn't match what he believes to be his skill set. One way of dealing with such a perception of a mismatch is the elusive behaviour you have indicated. These bees operate on the fringes as a means of survival.'

'That actually makes a lot of sense.'

'Over time the bees he works with begin to see him as fake and ineffective which can trigger a downward spiral in a bee who already lacks confidence.'

'And your prescription, doctor?' Dar Bee teased.

Bob Bee ignored the jibe and continued, 'Well, I think you must make a decision as to whether you believe Bogus Bee has the skill sets to add value to the hive.'

'I believe he does,' she replied immediately.

'Then we owe it to him to place him where his skill sets match and where he can add value. We also owe it to him to inform him of how he has been perceived and that we expect honesty and authenticity from him in the future.'

With a hint of defensiveness, Dar Bee asked, 'And what does Bogus Bee owe us? You make it sound like the issue lies with the management and not him.

'A management opportunity, my dear Dar Bee! A management opportunity!' he expostulated. 'Don't get me wrong. Bogus Bee must own his behaviour in the future. He certainly has the lion's share of responsibility. Do you remember my conversation with J. Bee?'

'Certainly.'

'So, you remember how we talked about choosing our attitudes?'

'I do.'

'The same principle applies here. Once we have helped Bogus Bee understand the gap in his current behaviour, and pointed him in a direction to match his skill sets with the hive's needs, well then, he gets to choose.'

'Choose his attitude?'

'Oh yes, awareness then attitude. The choice of attitude always follows awareness,' Bob Bee said knowingly. 'But then he must choose his behaviour one opportunity at a time.'

He could tell that Dar Bee did not grasp the full meaning of his words. 'The way Bogus Bee has historically behaved has been successful for him and has become a habit. In other words, his choices of behaviour have slipped to his subconscious. He likely doesn't really think about it.'

'Makes sense.'

'I believe that successfully changing behaviour requires keeping a high degree of consciousness and vigilance around behaviour opportunities. It is too easy to slip back to old habits.' Patting his notebook, he added, 'I have a little BEE acronym I use.

B *is for Become Aware*
E *is for Embrace Attitude*
E *is for Elect Actions*'

'You are so creative,' Dar Bee said. 'I will spend some time with Bogus Bee and see if I can use this to help him.'

As Dar Bee was leaving, she whispered, 'To Bee or not to Bee.'

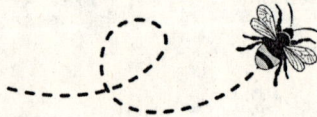

Bee a Great Communicator

Bee Attitude #6

'Communication is a skill that you can learn. It's like riding a bicycle or typing. If you're willing to work at it, you can rapidly improve the quality of every part of your life.'

—BRIAN TRACY

'Buzzda, buzzda, buzzda,' Gab Bee said as she chewed on a beeswax cud. There was no clear indication as to for whom the message was intended. This behaviour, however, was not unusual for Gab Bee. That is what she did. She talked and she talked and she talked... Dar Bee had done her best for years to try to manage her. Gab Bee was a worker bee and, by and large, she was a fairly productive bee.

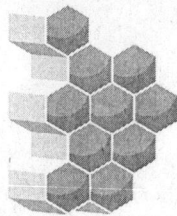

Hovering in front of Bob Bee's hexa-desk, Dar Bee said, 'You were exactly right, Bob Bee. The stress of this pollen and nectar shortage has certainly exacerbated some behaviours.'

Bob Bee peered over his little spectacles to suggest that he was listening. She then proceeded, saying, 'For example, in section eight I have a bee that talks all of the time. Historically, her incessant jabbering has been benign enough…'

'But now?'

'Now, she just talks about the increased workload, the longer hours, how tired she is, how much she misses her family. The list goes on.' She looked at Bob Bee with a pleading look.

'And how are the other bees responding to her?' Bob Bee asked.

'I see some of the bees rolling their eyes. Others just shake their heads. More than once I have heard bees say, "This is just how Gab Bee is." But it is having an effect on a few of the bees. They are joining in her banter, and I can see the morale deteriorating.' In exasperation, she buzzed, 'What do you think I should do Bob Bee?'

Bob Bee saw this situation as an opportunity to share another one of his Bee Attitudes. He said, 'Dar Bee, would you agree that in our colony it is important for the leaders, the managers and the frontline workers to be good communicators?'

Knowing Bob Bee and how often he asked questions for which the obvious answer was not always the best answer, she hesitantly replied, 'Well, yeeeessss?'

She was relieved when he said, 'I absolutely agree.' Then he added, 'And how would you define communication?'

A bit surprised by the question, she asked, 'What?'

'Communication. I want your definition of communication. It is a broad and ubiquitous term, but, at the core, what does it mean to you?'

Dar Bee thought for a few moments and then said, 'Communication is talking, listening, sharing thoughts and ideas.' She paused and then added, 'Also, understanding. Communication also includes understanding.'

She looked at Bob Bee expectantly.

Bob Bee smiled. 'Well, you certainly know the core elements of communication,' he offered.

'I do?' Dar Bee asked, smiling back.

'You do. But perhaps you will allow me to add a bit of structure and context to your definition?' he asked.

'Certainly!' Dar Bee replied, pulling out her little diary to take notes. 'I am sensing another Bee Attitude in the works.'

'Well,' Bob Bee said, stammering a bit. 'Well, yes. We have already established that being a good communicator is important in every role. Let me offer an alternative to your definition of communication.'

'Sure.'

'Not that your definition is necessarily wrong and mine is right. Let's be clear on that. What if we said that good communication is the exchange of accurate meaning between two or more bees?' He paused to allow her time to consider and then continued, 'Not just the exchange of words, not just the exchange of ideas but the exchange of the *real* meaning of the message each party wants to convey.'

'Yes!' Dar Bee said. 'I like that definition.'

'You know, you included "understanding" as part of your definition and for you that may represent what I am calling meaning.'

'I think you are right, but I think that the exchange of meaning is a bit more exacting,' she said.

'Good,' he said. 'Let's go one step further. In every communication event, there is a sender, a message, one or more receivers of the message and a feedback loop.'

Bob Bee then pulled out a sheet of paper and made a drawing of what he was trying to say.

The Communication Cycle

1 SENDER

2 MESSAGE

3 RECEIVER

4 FEEDBACK LOOP

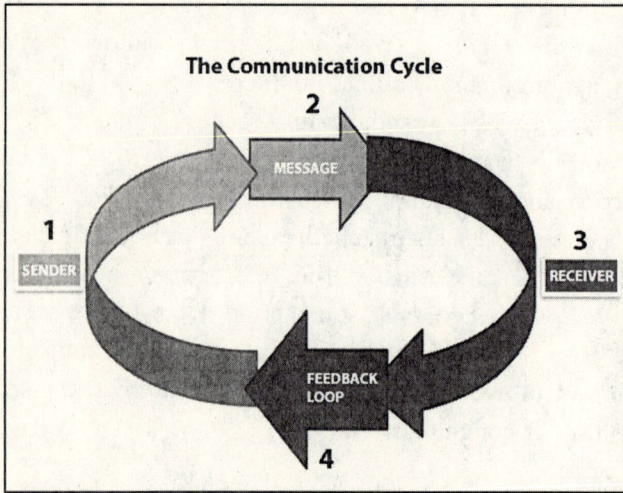

Dar Bee looked at the drawing and said, 'It's a circle.'

Bob Bee chuckled and stated, 'It is a circle, and the circle represents a cycle.'

Dar Bee gave him a questioning look.

Pointing at the drawing, Bob Bee said, 'The sender sends a message to one or more receivers.'

'Got it!'

'The message is then interpreted by the receiver.'

'Yes.'

'The receiver then sends back a message through the feedback loop to complete the cycle. The premise is that the receiver responds to the message in a way that signals to the sender that the meaning of the sender's message was interpreted correctly. See?'

'It just can't be that simple,' Dar Bee said sceptically.

Bob Bee laughed.

'Such a wise bee you are to be so young. Before, when I said "complete the cycle", I should have said "complete the *first* cycle." Often, we have to go through many cycles around this circle to arrive at clarity of meaning. There are two areas of focus here,' he said, adding a few more elements to the drawing. 'We must be intent on consistent clarity of our message, and we must practice true listening. We generally consider the sender as the one who originates the message, but as the cycle repeats itself you can see that both the participants alternate between being the sender and the receiver, and both have equal responsibility to promote consistent clarity and true listening.'

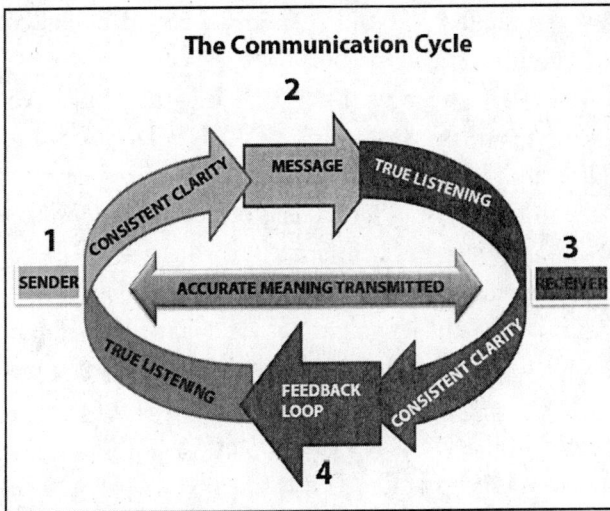

The Communication Cycle

'Thank you, Bob Bee. That is very helpful. Do you think you could guide me through how I can apply this with my "talker"?'

'I will try,' Bob Bee responded. 'What is her name?'

'Gab Bee.'

'Well, you might think that I should start with Gab Bee's communication style, but I want to take a step back from that. Tell me, Dar Bee, what has been your specific communication with Gab Bee about this issue; that is that you believe her communication is causing the deterioration of morale in some of her peers.'

Dar Bee was a bit stunned by the specificity of the question. 'Well, I have talked to her,' she began. 'I told her she was talking too much about negative stuff and she needed to lighten up.'

'And did that change her communication, her behaviour?'

Dar Bee smiled and said, 'Obviously not or I wouldn't be in here discussing it with you.'

'I would encourage you to go back to her and have the discussion again. But first think through what you want her to understand. Is it that she needs to "lighten up" or that you are seeing morale issues with some of her colleagues because of her negative communication? And is it that you need her to communicate to others in a way that is supportive of the team during this challenging time? And is it that if she needs to vent or to make suggestions, your door is always open?'

Dar Bee let out a sigh. 'So, you are saying that Gab Bee's communication issue is my issue, right?'

'What I am saying Dar Bee is that we all—Gab Bee, you, me, Queen Bee—have responsibility for how we communicate and how we behave. My point is that your first responsibility is to look in the mirror and make sure that you have done all you can do to transmit true meaning in your communication before you start judging others.'

Dar Bee considered. Finally, she said, 'That's fair.'

'Just to be clear, I am not suggesting that you back up on your expectations. Just make sure they are clear.' Bob Bee paused and then added, 'And once you begin that communication cycle, remember the feedback loop and practise true listening. If I have learnt anything over the years, it is that sometimes those we see as dissenters or having behavioural issues, often have a lot of value to add. While you were talking, I thumbed through the productivity reports and Gab Bee is consistently at the top of her department. Perhaps, you can move the conversation to that topic and see if she has insights or suggestions for the rest of the department.'

On the way back to her department, Dar Bee began to fully digest the conversation that she had just had with Bob Bee. She said to herself, 'I cannot necessarily control others' communication and behaviour, but I can control my own. When I do that, I, at least, may influence theirs.'

Bob Bee had come a long way in the area of communication, but he knew he could still improve. He had recently read a book called *What I Really Meant to Say!* which had guidance that went from A to Z. He felt that it provided great direction on communication. He also felt that the instruction there was a good primer to represent communication in his Bee Attitudes.

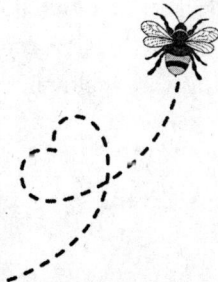

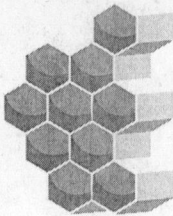

Bee Curious

Bee Attitude #7

'Curiosity is the engine of achievement'

—KEN ROBINSON

'Why do they call him Sweat Bee?' Bob Bee asked. Dar Bee smiled. 'It's just a nickname he got when he first got here.'

Bob Bee gestured for her to continue.

'Well, when he first came on, he asked so many questions that his boss told him that he was making him sweat with all his questions.'

Bob Bee looked at his personnel file and said, 'It looks like Sweat Bee has done well in such a short period of time.'

'He has,' Dar Bee replied. 'That is why I brought him to your attention. I wanted to know if he meets the criteria to be included in your Bee Attitudes.'

With dramatic flair, Bob Bee pulled out his notebook and began turning the pages. 'Let's see. Let's see,' he said with an exaggerated tone. 'Well, this might be a fit. But I will need to ask you a few questions?'

'Ask away,' Dar Bee said.

'First, what was the nature of his questions?'

Dar Bee became thoughtful. Finally, she said, 'Well, like I said, there were multiple questions, but they were mostly questions about what his role was, what were the expectations from him. You know, questions like that.'

'Thank you,' Bob Bee said. 'Second, what was his attitude as he asked the questions?'

'Attitude? I am not really sure what you mean.'

'Let's see,' Bob Bee said, trying to reframe the question. 'What did you perceive to be his disposition as he asked these questions. I mean, was he asking them like he was a know-it-all and was trying to catch someone saying something wrong? Was he trying to be the centre of attention, or did he seem like he was really interested in understanding the answers?'

'The last one, like he was really interested in understanding the answers. Remember, I wasn't actually there. I am just responding to your questions based on what his supervisor told me.'

Bob Bee considered and then asked, 'Did his supervisor seem to be irritated with him for being so inquisitive?'

'No,' Dar Bee replied definitively. 'It was kind of funny, you know. He was a seasoned supervisor and told me that the questions actually got him thinking about how his department was conducting business.'

Bob Bee smiled. He pulled out his notebook again and turned the pages. 'Well, Dar Bee,' he said, as if conducting a ceremony, 'you have presented a qualified candidate to the membership of the Bee Attitudes...'

Dar Bee bowed.

After a dramatic pause, Bob Bee said, '...Bee Curious.'

'Bee Curious?'

'Yes, Bee Curious,' answered Bob Bee. 'As simple as it may sound, the bees who seem to excel ask a lot of questions. They want to understand how things work, how they fit in and ultimately how they can get better at what they do.'

'That actually does sound simple,' Dar Bee offered.

'But I want you to think about the questions that I just asked you. The supervisor told you that Sweat Bee's questions were not irritating.'

'Yes.'

'That speaks to the spirit of the questions. If Sweat Bee was asking the questions to seek attention or to show off repeatedly, well, that would quickly become irritating and cause the supervisor to shut down or react in some other way. Instead, it actually inspired the supervisor.'

Dar Bee nodded and said, 'So, the curiosity should manifest itself in a spirit of respect?'

'You got it!' Bob Bee exclaimed.

Dar Bee was thoughtful. Finally, she said, 'You know, I understand a New Bee having a lot of questions. She is just getting used to her job. How does this work? How does that work? What do I do if this happens?'

'Naturally,' Bob Bee agreed.

'But the more seasoned bee should know the answers to those types of questions, right?'

'I absolutely agree with you,' Bob Bee grinned, and continued, 'And the more seasoned bee should have more seasoned questions.'

Dar Bee cocked her head questioningly.

'In the spirit of change, improvement, progress if you will, our bees should maintain a healthy level of curiosity. The bee that has been around longer will have more experience and more context, so it is likely that their questions may be more sophisticated. And whether it is with their supervisor, in a departmental meeting or some other forum, we should promote a culture that allows for these questions.'

'As long as they are asked in a respectful manner,' Dar Bee added.

'Correct, as long as they are asked in a respectful manner.'

Dar Bee looked at Bob Bee's wingpack. Noticing this, he promptly said, 'Yes, I will be adding some action items to my Bee Attitudes tonight.'

They both laughed.

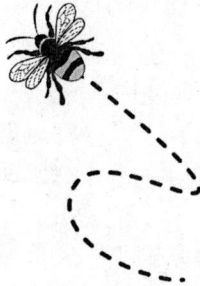

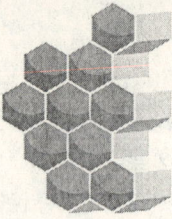

Bee Frank

Bee Attitude #8

'Frankness is not a license to say anything you want, wherever and whenever you want. It is not rudeness.'

—RICK WARREN

'Frank Bee had come a long way. There was a time when many would say they were put off by Frank Bee's directness. Others would get downright angry with him and go out of their way to avoid him,' Bob Bee was explaining to Dar Bee.

Frank Bee had long retired, but Bob Bee knew his story well and believed it very important to pass on the story of the importance of being frank.

'I've got a few employees like him,' Dar Bee said. 'They are a mixed bag.'

Bob Bee cocked his head with a questioning look on his face.

'What I mean is when they speak candidly, they often raise important issues or opportunities that might otherwise go unnoticed.'

'Ah, yes!' Bob Bee replied knowingly, 'But?'

'Yes…but is right,' she acknowledged. 'But they seem to

have a way of rubbing bees the wrong way,' Dar Bee added, rubbing her wings together. 'There ought to be a happy medium, you know? How do we go about training bees to speak openly and honestly, but to do so in a way that is not so abrasive?'

'Now that is absolutely the honey question right there, Dar Bee. I'm not sure there is a singular answer to the question, but I can tell you what happened to Frank Bee.'

'Do tell!' Dar Bee replied with interest.

'Well, Frank Bee's openness was a novelty to management and even his staff for a while. His hive had become used to talking around issues and challenges and so when Frank Bee came along and began "calling it like he saw it", his style was initially seen as refreshing.'

'I have a feeling here comes the "but",' Dar Bee put in with a smile.

'Yes. But he did not balance his frankness with kindness. The novelty of being frank soon wore off. His leaders and peers saw him as an arrogant know-it-all instead. Unbeknownst to him, he was on a downward spiral, until…'

'Until you counselled him?' Dar Bee asked.

Smiling, Bob Bee stated, 'Well, it wasn't me. But luckily for Frank Bee, some bee did pull him aside privately and helped him understand how he was coming across to others.'

'And he changed?'

'He did. He did indeed! Frank Bee was, like most bees, a good bee with good intentions. So, after he understood the negative perceptions he was creating, it wasn't a stretch for him to remind himself that he could be respectful of others without watering down his opinions. And you know what follows respectfulness?' Bob Bee asked wryly.

Dar Bee had known Bob Bee long enough to understand that this was a rhetorical question. She waited silently until he finally offered, 'Kindness, that's what serial respectfulness leads to. Frank Bee did not stop telling it the way he saw it. What changed was the way he told it. He became more selective with his audience. He began to have many of his conversations privately. His tone softened. His word choice was more deliberate, more encouraging. He began to focus his message on the process that was in question and did not put the focus on the people.'

'Amazing,' Dar Bee interjected.

'Amazing is exactly the word some of his colleagues used to describe the change. Over time, the change in his style led to a high level of trust from his peers.'

'It looks like you may have learnt a thing or two from Frank Bee,' Dar Bee said coyly.

'Huh?'

'You are always frank with me, but you are never unkind.'

She thought she saw Bob Bee blush a little.

'With this new stressor, we will need to perhaps give little guidance to those who have a disposition of directness,' Bob Bee said.

Dar Bee responded, 'I think we can tell them the story of the importance of being frank. If that doesn't inspire them, nothing will.'

'I will go one flight further.'

'One flight further than what?' Dar Bee asked, confused.

'One flight further than telling the story,' he said. 'I looked up Frank Bee and he has agreed to meet with a few of the direct bees who could use his guidance.'

'That is amazing. I can give you three names off the top of my head.'

'You ask a few questions and get the list together. I will arrange for him to be here next week, and I will ask him to be on the lookout for some new guidance that we might put in our Bee Attitudes.'

'So now they are *our* Bee Attitudes, are they? I haven't seen the entire list yet,' Dar Bee teased.

'Patience, my dear friend. I promise you will see it soon enough.'

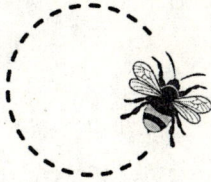

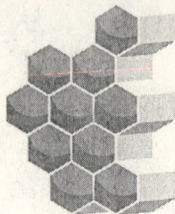

Bee Kind

Bee Attitude #9

'You cannot do kindness to soon, for
you never know how soon it will be too late.'

—RALPH WALDO EMERSON

Dar Bee hovered in the background and watched Phil Bee do what he did best, with admiration. Phil Bee had been in her department for a number of years and he, more than any of her other bees, seemed to be tuned into the feelings of the bees.

Privately, Dar Bee was a bit jealous of Phil's intuitiveness. She saw herself as a logical bee, but not without consideration for others' feelings. She had noticed more than once that when she had delivered a message to her bees that was in the 'difficult message' category, some of the bees had shot furtive looks towards Phil.

Now, he was helping a New Bee adjust to some of the new pressures of the work. She listened to their conversation:

Phil Bee: 'I understand that it takes some adjustments to get it right. We are all going through a learning curve.'

New Bee: 'I feel like I understand the overall process, but I seem to be making the same mistakes over and over.'

Phil Bee: 'You know, I have been having the same issues. Why don't we do a few cycles together and see if we can keep each other on track?'

New Bee: 'That would be great!'

Dar Bee watched as Phil Bee politely guided New Bee through the work process. New Bee was, in fact, making some very fundamental errors and Phil Bee quietly showed the former his mistake, how to correct it and how to avoid making it again in the next cycle. Dar Bee could not hear everything that was being said, but she could see that the New Bee was shaking his head up and down and smiling intermittently. In the wake of the recent conversation about Frank Bee and how his disposition had migrated towards kindness, Dar Bee was impressed with Phil Bee.

After New Bee was gone, Dar Bee buzzed over to Phil Bee and said, 'I don't know how you do it.'

Phil Bee replied innocently, 'Do what?'

'You are always so kind to everyone. I have heard the humans say that you catch more flies with honey. Is that what makes you so kind?' Dar Bee inquired.

Phil Bee frowned. 'And just why would they want more flies?' he asked.

'Oh, I think it is just one of their sayings. I think it means that they will get more of what they want from others if they are nice instead of being mean.'

Phil Bee considered. Finally, he said, 'No, I choose to be kind because I believe it is the right thing to do.'

Dar Bee was silent. After a few moments, Phil Bee added, 'Don't get me wrong. I do believe that is the probable outcome; that is, that bees prefer other bees being nice and the result is generally more often positive than when a bee shows a negative or mean spirit.'

'I agree,' Dar Bee interjected.

'But I...'

Dar Bee sensed that Phil Bee was having an internal struggle as to what to say next or whether to say anything at all.

Finally, Phil Bee said, 'This is very personal for me. You see, my father was not a nice bee. I saw him being mean to his friends and family, including me sometimes. I didn't like what I saw, and I told myself at a very young age that I would not be like that. But with the pressures that came with growing into an adult bee, I found myself sliding towards responding to others with sarcasm and, well, sometimes just downright meanness.'

He looked at Dar Bee as if in pain.

'I understand,' she said with sympathy.

'At one point, I thought my disposition was genetic. My father was not a nice bee; therefore, I would not be a nice bee either.'

There was a long pause as Phil Bee stared past Dar Bee.

Dar Bee broke the silence, saying, 'But something must have happened. You are one of the kindest bees I know.'

Phil Bee's eyes met hers. 'Yes, something happened that changed my life. A colleague, a good friend, pulled me aside one day after watching me go on a tirade about something at work. He had known me for years and knew my dad as well. He went on to say something like this to me, "I have seen a change in you over the past few years. You are not your father. You are Phil Bee. Your thoughts and your actions are yours. How you talk to others, how you treat others is your choice. It was not passed to you through your father's DNA.

'"When you become irritated or angry, some aspects of your needs are not being met. That can happen at home or at work. Maybe the other person or persons you are dealing with did something wrong, made an error or behaved badly according to your standards. You can continue down this path of lashing out at them. However, I can tell you that that often does not end well.

'"You can make the choice—and yes, Phil Bee, it is a choice—you can make the choice to respond to others with kindness to try to remedy the wrong, correct the mistake or change the behaviour. Go home tonight and look in the mirror. Ask yourself what kind of bee would you want to be."'

'And that was when you changed?' Dar Bee asked.

'That is when I started my journey,' Phil Bee replied. 'It didn't happen overnight, but I began to understand that how I responded and communicated with others was really my choice. As I began to constructively act on that, my life began to change. I still have a lot to learn.'

'I think there is a lot you can teach me and others,' Dar Bee said.

'Perhaps,' Phil Bee replied. 'I do know this though. It costs very little to be kind to others. For those you are kind to, though, the dividends can be tremendous.'

'Well said. Well said, indeed.'

Dar Bee made a note to talk to Bob Bee. If being kind was not on his Bee Attitude list, she would encourage him to add it.

Later, she was happy to learn that it was definitely on his list. From what she had learnt from Phil Bee, she was confident she could add some points to the action items once she had a chance to see it.

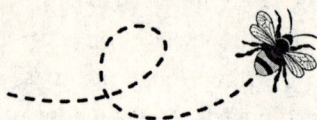

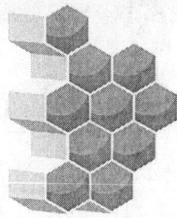

Bee Humble

Bee Attitude #10

'What is most needed for learning is a humble mind.'

—CONFUCIUS

Humble Bee was well respected by everyone in the colony. Well, there were perhaps those few bees who did not necessarily like Humble Bee, but Dar Bee put that down to envy.

Humble Bee was a team player. When the Queen Bee had made the announcement about flying further and working harder to meet production, Humble Bee was the first one in the subsequent departmental meeting to offer suggestions about tactical strategies. And she wasn't one of those bees, like Bogus Bee, who offered recommendations, but then would fly away and let the other bees do the work. Even for the work, she was the first in line.

It was clear, however, that Humble Bee wasn't looking for recognition or credit. With her language, her tone, her timing, her choice of words, somehow, she was able to engage the other bees in productive conversations and actions without drawing attention to herself.

Dar Bee pulled her aside one afternoon and asked if they could talk for a few minutes.

'Absolutely!' Humble Bee answered. 'Always glad to catch up.'

They found a quiet place and Dar Bee said, 'You are one of the most unassuming bees I have ever met.'

Humble Bee blushed.

'And yet, I see the respect your peers have for you. Frankly, I am in awe of your disposition, the way you handle yourself.' She paused before finally asking, 'Have you always been like this?'

'Well, you might not believe this,' Humble Bee began quietly, 'but at one time I was quite the arrogant bee.'

'No!' Dar Bee responded emphatically.

'It's true. It was another place and time but, yes, back then certainly no one would call me unassuming.'

Before Dar Bee could ask, Humble Bee added, 'And you might have the question of what happened? What changed me?'

Dar Bee shook her head in affirmation.

Humble Bee looked off into the distance and then said, 'I can't name an exact time or even an exact event that changed me. What I can tell you is that one day I came to the understanding about myself; that I am a part of something bigger.' She looked at Dar Bee, then smiled and continued, 'Now, I am not getting all metaphysical on you. It was nothing like that. It was just that I came to a realization that I have a place, a role if you will, at home and at work and that I didn't always have to be the centre of attention or in control.' Meeting Dar Bee's eyes, she asked, 'Do you understand?'

'I think so,' Dar Bee replied.

'I must say, it was a bit of a surprise for me that as I began to give credit to others, as I tried to put others' wants and needs in the forefront, as I began to work on truly listening, well...it was quite freeing,' Humble Bee said with a smile.

'Freeing? How so?' Dar Bee inquired.

Humble Bee considered and then said, 'I think it was because before I was so self-reliant, you know? I felt the weight of what needed to be done on my wings. When I started sharing that load with my co-workers and my family in certain situations, I realized that...' she stopped and Dar Bee realized she was blushing again.

'You realized what?' Dar Bee urged.

'You will laugh at me,' Humble Bee said shyly.

Putting a wing over her heart, Dar Bee said, 'I promise not to laugh.'

'Well,' Humble Bee began speaking again after some hesitation, 'I realized that what I came to know as the "We Bee" has more strength, more intellect, more resilience than the "Me Bee".' 'And that...' she added with zeal, 'that was quite freeing.'

'It seems that you traded arrogance for humility,' Dar Bee offered.

'You say "traded". That word might be a bit too strong. It seems to imply a transaction, that is, it seems to suggest that I give something and I get something. It happened with much more subtlety than that.'

She chuckled, then said, 'It was more evolutionary than revolutionary. I certainly had to work on it. I had to maintain vigilance on my desire to control and manage everything.'

She paused and seemed to look past Dar Bee. She then said, 'But over time, the need to be at the centre of everything has been superseded by the need to contribute in a meaningful way.'

Dar Bee could tell that Humble Bee was deciding whether to talk further. Finally, Humble Bee said, 'I tend to believe that this style that I have developed, what you are calling humility, I believe it is particularly good for our New Bees.'

'How so?' Dar Bee asked with interest.

'Well, these New Bees, they are young and ready to conquer the world. They are educated and certainly most of them are very bright.'

She paused and then said, 'But they lack experience, you know. Their preparation in school is certainly needed but there is always a gap between the theories they learn and the real-life day-to-day activity of the hive.'

'There is no doubt about that,' Dar Bee interjected.

'They need, what should I call it? They need a buffer. Someone who can ease them into the realities of the hive without stifling that authentic, pent-up energy.' She was thoughtful, then said, 'We won't mention names here, but if we were to connect these New Bees with mentors who throw these bees to the bears instead of nurturing that energy and flying that tightrope, well our turnover rate would be much higher.'

Dar Bee smiled and said, 'With your permission, I would like to tell Bob Bee about our conversation. He is working on a list of behaviours that he believes contributes to the success of our colony and I think humility should be on that list.'

Humble Bee prepared her wings to leave. Smiling, she said, 'You can certainly tell him about the conversation but maybe you could leave my name out of it.' As she flew off, Humble Bee looked back and winked at Dar Bee.

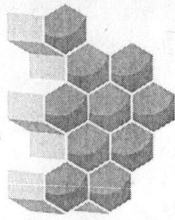

Bee Ambitious

Bee Attitude #11

'Without ambition one starts nothing.
Without work, one finishes nothing.
The prize will not be sent to you.
You have to win it.'

—RALPH WALDO EMERSON

'But you just talked about being humble and now you are saying that "Bee Ambitious" is on the list of Bee Attitudes?' Dar Bee asked Bob Bee incredulously.

It was, in fact, just one day after they had discussed the quality of humility and Bob Bee had agreed that 'Bee Humble' should definitely be on the list. Then, without hesitation, he had blurted out that 'Bee Ambitious' was the next Bee Attitude on the list.

'That is exactly what I am saying,' Bob Bee said with an air of pride.

'But that doesn't make sense to me. Isn't that counterintuitive?'

Bob Bee smiled and said, 'I was exactly like you the first time I thought through this. What I came to realize, however, is that the two, humility and ambition, what shall I call them…?'

'Attitudes. Bee Attitudes,' Dar Bee put in, smirking and pointing at the notebook.

'Oh yes. Attitudes. How silly of me. These two attitudes are not mutually exclusive. Many bees do not like the concept of being ambitious because it has a stigma attached to it.'

Dar Bee nodded in agreement.

'But that is because,' Bob Bee continued, 'thoughts of ambition connote the idea of competing against other bees. The stigma often lends itself to a win-lose proposition. If one bee wins, then another bee loses. One bee gets the promotion. Another bee does not get it. You agree?' Bob Bee asked enthusiastically.

'Wholeheartedly!' Dar Bee replied.

'But what if we reframed our definition of being ambitious around the idea of competing against yourself, not others?' Bob Bee asked in a professorial attitude.

'Go on,' Dar Bee urged.

'For example, we all have work goals, right? We are to contribute to produce X amount of honey in Y amount of time frame?'

'Yes.'

'What if a bee who wants to get better at something establishes his or her own goals but, by and large, keeps the aspiration to themselves.'

'Explain!' Dar Bee demanded with a smile.

'Suppose, a bee wanted to understand how the bee supply chain works. Her current job is very task-specific. She believes that a broader understanding of the supply chain will enhance her skills and perhaps make her better at her job. She is interested in bettering herself. She is not necessarily vying for an immediate promotion nor is she practising a one-upbeeship on her peers. Does she think the increased knowledge would be helpful to her in the trajectory of her career? Perhaps. But she is not taking supply chain night classes to be better than another bee. She is taking the classes to better herself. And only the closest of her bee friends know that she is doing it.'

'So,' Dar Bee said knowingly, 'it seems that ambition is defined by whether a bee is trying to better him or herself for personal reasons versus competing with other bees.'

Bob Bee considered. 'The way you put it certainly gets to the crux of my definition of ambition. But our world is not that simple, is it?'

'No. No, it's not,' Dar Bee replied.

'Perhaps,' Bob Bee offered, 'it may be helpful to look at the broader characteristics of ambitious bees to better understand why I have "Bee Ambitious" on my list.'

Pulling out her diary, Dar Bee said, 'Ready!'

'For starters,' Bob Bee replied quickly, 'bees that are ambitious are open-minded. They don't think they know it all and they are willing to learn from others.'

'Check,' Dar Bee said, finishing her note.

'Second, ambitious bees are quite good at setting goals and then listing the action steps to reach their goals.'

'Check!'

Bob Bee considered, then said, 'I should have shared this first. Ambitious bees are always trying to improve themselves.'

'Got it. Next?' Dar Bee asked.

'Ambitious bees are not afraid to fail. In fact, they expect to fail some to be ultimately successful.'

'Wow!' Dar Bee put in.

'Wow is right. And they are also very self-aware,' Bob Bee added. By the frown on Dar Bee's face, Bob Bee knew he needed to provide a little more explanation for this one. 'Do you remember I said they compete against themselves, not other bees?'

'Yes.'

'While they know that, ambitious bees are very aware that other bees may not perceive their desires and actions as selfless. In fact, they know that some bees may be a little threatened by their ambition. Ambitious bees don't want that kind of reaction, but they are quite aware it can exist. Thus, they go out of their way to be discreet.'

'Got it,' Dar Bee said. 'That makes sense. Anything else?'

Bob Bee checked his own notebook. After a few moments, he said, 'This goes without saying but just in case. Ambitious bees are willing to take on a challenge. They stay positive and focus on achieving goals but...'

Dar Bee added the last part of the sentence, 'But not at the expense of other bees.'

'You got it!' Bob Bee replied. 'Not at the expense of other bees.'

Wryly, Dar Bee said, 'When I finally do get a comprehensive look at that list, I bet I can add a few action items in this category.'

'No doubt you can,' Bob Bee said over his wing as he flew off.

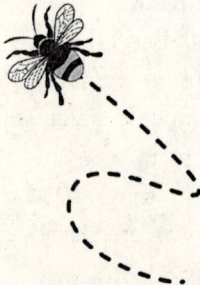

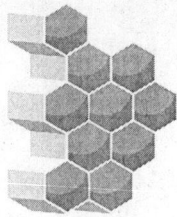

Bee a Team Player

Bee Attitude #12

'Teams are incredible things. No task is too great, no accomplishment too grand, no dream too far-fetched for a team. It takes teamwork to make the dream work.'

—JOHN C. MAXWELL

Just as in stressful circumstances in the past, a few bees had cut and flown after the Queen Bee had made her announcement. They thought the honey was golder on the other side of the orchard. But none of the bees in the nectar division had left.

A great number of bees worked in this department which retrieved and managed the nectar. And this was no easy task. The nectar is not only the main ingredient for the honey, but also the main source of energy for the bees. The bees suck up the droplets of nectar from the flowers, and swallow it to break down the complex sugars into more simple sugars. Once they get back to the colony, they pass it along to the 'house' bees who take it inside and pack it away in the hexagon-shaped beeswax cells. Then, the bees use their wings to create a warm breeze and dry out the nectar, which turns it to honey.

Given the shortage of nearby nectar and how critical it

was for the bees' survival, any reasonable bee might have expected a lot of turnover in this area. But other than planned retirements, there were no turnovers in this department. Dar Bee was interested to see if she could learn something from these bees that she could then pass on to other departments. She asked their manager if she could meet with a bee or two and the manager was happy to comply but with the caveat that her bees could not be gone away from their work for too long under the current circumstances.

Dar Bee hovered across the small conference room table with a bee hovering and staring politely back at her. She began, 'Hello, I'm Dar Bee. Did your manager explain why I wanted to talk with you?'

'She did,' the bee replied shyly.

'And you are?' Dar Bee urged.

'Oh, please pardon my manners,' he responded, 'I am Lowell Bee.'

'Nice to meet you,' Dar Bee replied with a nod. Without further ado, she continued, 'I am hoping to learn anything I can from you that might help us understand the high degree of loyalty in this department compared to some others. Even in trying times, your department seems to maintain high productivity, quality and employee satisfaction scores and no bees seem to quit or even transfer to another department. What are your thoughts, Lowell Bee?'

Lowell Bee put a wing under his chin and became pensive. After several moments he looked up and said, 'If I had to point to one thing...'

He paused for effect, and then continued, 'Well, I couldn't say it was just one thing.' He chuckled at his own joke and Dar Bee joined in. He added, 'You do understand that you are talking to a mere "house" bee, right?'

Dar Bee smiled and said, 'Take the word "mere" out of that sentence and I will reply with a resounding "yes". I know you work hard on the frontlines. I know that the frontline is where many of our challenges lie. But I also know that it is where many of our opportunities and solutions are as well. To be clear, I believe the Queen Bee, the drones, the house bees, all the different bees have different roles, but I do not believe one is better or more important than the other. Also, I think that sometimes our management does not always communicate their trust in the frontline bees who offer new ideas or bring solutions to our challenges and issues.'

'You've hit the proboscis on the pistil!' Lowell Bee exclaimed.

'What?' Dar Bee reacted in surprise.

'What you just said; that is, that you believe all of us have different roles but that we are equal, and we are all important,' Lowell offered.

'Yes,' urged Dar Bee.

'That's exactly what our manager believes,' he said with a sudden onset of pride. 'And I believe that is the foundation to the answer you are seeking.'

'Can you elaborate?' Dar Bee encouraged.

'I have worked in colonies where management tells you what to do, when to do and how to do. So, you just do it. There was little time for questions or suggestions from the house bees,' he began. 'But here, at least in our department, our manager takes time for those questions and suggestions. She, in fact, encourages them. We meet at least once a week, more if needed and she tries to keep us informed about what is going on across the colony. She treats the bees fairly.'

He paused, and then said, 'Now, don't get me wrong. Her expectations of work ethic, quality and service are high, but she matches that with respect. She respects us.'

'That type of respect goes a long way,' Dar Bee encouraged.

'It does,' Lowell Bee responded enthusiastically. 'A bee doesn't mind flying the extra mile when needed when you work for a bee like that. I have a hunch that a few bees make a habit of switching colonies for more honey, but my guess is that most bees leave because of their relationship with their supervisor.'

They were both silent for a moment. Dar Bee was surprised at the depth of insight Lowell Bee gave in what he said next: 'I am, for some reason, drawn to the nature versus nurture debate. I believe that most bees begin with an intrinsic tendency, at least on some level, to be loyal. For the work setting, that initial loyalty is enmeshed in the implied compact of the agreement between the bee and the colony.'

Moving one wing to the other and back, he said in a mock professional voice, 'I will give you X amount of honey and you will give me Y amount of work.' Then, switching back to his normal voice, he added, 'The agreement is transactional.' He looked at Dar Bee to see if she was following.

She nodded.

'This initial agreement baselines the loyalty, then the nurture part takes over,' he said knowingly. 'The things we talked about—listening, respect, fair treatment, keeping connected to the rest of the organization, how well these are done—well that determines whether the loyalty grows, stagnates or goes in the other direction.'

'You seem wise beyond your years,' Dar Bee said earnestly.

'Well, I don't know about that,' Lowell Bee replied, blushing a little.

'Anything else to help me understand loyalty?' Dar Bee inquired.

'Just one thing,' Lowell Bee answered seriously. 'It might be easy to assume that the way I have communicated my thoughts on loyalty, that management has the primary responsibility for nurturing it. However, I believe the bees in my department know that the nurturing goes both ways.'

Dar Bee urged him to explain.

'Well, we understand that the colony has finite resources. We understand that our manager cannot make every one of our suggestions happen. We understand that there are times, like now, when we have to fly up and do more work. We don't berate our manager when these things happen. We support her because we know she has got our wings. It's a bit of give and take, isn't it?'

Dar Bee wanted to talk longer but honouring the manager's wishes, she thanked Lowell Bee for his time and valuable information. She had taken plenty of notes to add to the 'Bee a Team Player' Bee Attitude.

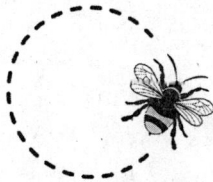

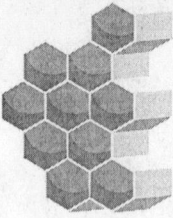

Bee Independent

Bee Attitude #13

'Diversity is the art of thinking independently together.'

—MALCOLM FORBES

D ar Bee had just finished telling Bob Bee about her conversation with Lowell Bee and how the department worked so well as a team, including the manager. As soon as she finished the story, she added emphatically, 'Being a team player is important, but we also need independent bees.'

'I think we have another case of seemingly diametrically opposed Bee Attitudes,' Bob Bee offered jokingly.

'"Diametrically opposed Bee Attitudes",' she said in a mocking manner. 'You are staying up at night and reading the dictionary again, aren't you?'

They both laughed.

'Now,' Dar Bee continued. 'Take Free Bee for example.'

'Free Bee?' Bob Bee asked.

'Yep!' With a faraway look in her eye, Dar Bee said, 'An old colleague of mine at a previous hive.'

'I thought this was the only hive you've worked at,' Bob Bee said incredulously.

Dar Bee gave him a wry smile. 'There might be a lot you don't know about me,' she replied.

'So, this Free Bee, he was an independent bee?' Bob Bee asked.

'She,' Dar Bee corrected him. 'And yes, she was. But just like the stigma you brought up with "Bee Ambitious", even "Bee Independent" carries a bit of a stigma.'

Bob Bee gave Dar Bee a salute with his wing and said, 'Now you are the teacher, and I am the student. I am ready to learn.'

'If you were talking with another bee at work who made a statement such as "that bee, he is such an independent bee", what would your gut reaction be?'

'Well,' Bob Bee replied, 'I would probably need a little more context and I would want to know the tone of the bee that was telling me this.'

'You are over-analysing it,' Dar Bee interrupted. 'Based on your experience—your gut—would you view this as a positive statement or a critical one?'

Bob Bee considered. Finally, he said, 'I would probably lean toward the idea that it was a critical statement.'

Appreciating his response, Dar Bee said, 'We work best as a team. Our roles are distinct but integrated to produce the honey for the hive. So, when we start thinking or talking about an independent bee, it causes us to mentally challenge the current process. If we have distinct roles in the hive and we understand that our roles integrate for the good of the hive, then the concept of an independent bee can create a cognitive dissonance in our mental model of how things are supposed to be.'

'Now who is staying up and perusing the dictionary?' Bob

Bee joked. 'Cognitive dissonance?' he asked.

Dar Bee blushed. Then she remembered that she had actually learnt this concept when Bob Bee was discussing Bogus Bee. 'I learnt that from you,' she said smugly.

'Did you now?'

'I did. Perhaps, the way you said it earlier, when you referred to Bee Humble and Bee Ambitious is a better way to describe what I am trying to say though. The idea of being humble and being ambitious are not mutually exclusive.'

'Got it,' Bob Bee offered.

'Well, it's the same with the idea of being a team player and being independent. They do not have to be mutually exclusive.'

Bob Bee pulled out his notebook and prepared to take notes.

'It might be helpful for me to tell you about Free Bee and why I believe she exemplifies the "Bee Independent" Bee Attitude.'

'Sounds good.'

'It's really a myriad of characteristics, you understand, that add up to the independence I am talking about,' Dar Bee said. 'And to be clear, some of what I am going to tell you is what I observed and some of it Free Bee and I actually discussed before I left that hive. I was intrigued by her, and I had a chance to hover with her and ask a few questions.'

Bob Bee indicated that he was listening.

'Well, the first characteristic of an independent bee, I would say, is a high level of self-awareness.'

Without looking up from his notebook, Bob Bee said, 'Meaning?'

'Well,' Dar Bee said thoughtfully, 'such a bee does not get

entangled in the politics or drama of the hive. There were a lot of internal politics and drama at play in the previous hive. While I found myself getting all worked up over some of these things, Free Bee always seemed to steer clear of the distractions that can accompany the machinations of the organization.'

'Interesting.'

'It wasn't that she was unaware of these things,' Dar Bee added. 'She just did not allow herself to become embroiled in them.'

'How do you think she managed that?' Bob Bee asked.

'I believe that she had a very good understanding of herself, you see. She knew her role. She understood her belief system. She knew what her knowledge base was. She kept her emotions in check. She was in touch with her basic assumptions, beliefs and biases.'

Bob Bee looked up. He said, 'These traits of Free Bee that you describe, they are certainly admirable. But I fail to make the connection to the idea of an independent bee.'

Dar Bee frowned. 'Will you allow me to continue to make my points?' she said, pretending to be hurt by his interruption.

Apologetically, Bob Bee gestured for her to continue.

'I believe it is this high level of self-awareness that is a precursor to being self-motivated,' Dar Bee said.

Sitting up a bit and leaning into Dar Bee, Bob Bee said, 'First you throw out cognitive dissonance at me and now the word precursor. I feel like I have missed a few days in school.'

'Again, you threw out cognitive dissonance first. And precursor. I believe you know exactly what that means.'

Bob Bee shrugged his wings.

'You know. One thing has to come before the other. For

example, you can't make honey without the nectar.'

Bob Bee nodded affirmatively.

'Well, you can't be an independent bee, well a successful independent bee at least, unless you have a high level of self-awareness.'

Playfully, Bob Bee said, 'And that leads you to the honey?'

'What it leads you to,' Dar Bee responded, 'is self-motivation.'

Bob Bee readied his pen again.

'You see, Free Bee, as I said, knew herself, her capabilities, her strengths and her weaknesses. She also kept in touch with the goals of the hive. And it was that platform of self-awareness that gave her the freedom to think and act independently.'

Bob Bee raised his eyes from his notebook and was about to speak but Dar Bee intervened.

In her feigned professorial voice she said, 'I am deducing…' she dramatically bowed to Bob Bee and said, '…that my learned colleague is about to inquire as to the level of risk of such independent thinking and acting.'

Bob Bee pretended to tip a cap on his head as a signal that she was spot on.

'As Free Bee so gracefully demonstrated to the hive, this idea of "independence" does not come without some restraint,' Dar Bee lectured. 'She simply did not require external forces for her to bring thoughts, ideas and action to the teams she was on and the hive she served. She still respected the team members and their roles. She did not fly by them disrespectfully. But she also didn't just buzz around and wait for someone to tell her what to do.'

'Do you have an example?' Bob Bee asked.

'I do,' Dar Bee replied without hesitation. 'This was a long time ago and we were experiencing a similar challenge to increase honey production. Free Bee was on the nectar retrieval team. There was some delay in the storage section resulting in some of the nectar being ruined before it could be stored. Free Bee called a meeting and proposed a staggered schedule for the bee retrieval team throughout the day, so that the arrival of the nectar occurred in a more metered fashion.'

'And it worked?'

'You bet it worked,' Dar Bee said proudly as if it were her own idea. 'The amazing thing is this. At the time, Free Bee was only in her third month of work.

'No!' Bob Bee exclaimed. 'A New Bee?'

'That's right. A New Bee. And, if I may, I will take you back to our core discussion. It was her understanding of herself, her self-awareness, coupled with her understanding of the needs of the hive that allowed this New Bee to undertake such a bold action.'

'And none of the other bees, the more seasoned ones, got upset?'

'They did not. Her independent thinking and actions were in alignment with the hive needs.'

'Suppose her recommendation was not accepted by the other bees or was accepted but not successful. Wouldn't that look bad for Free Bee?' Bob Bee questioned.

Dar Bee considered the question. 'I don't think so,' she replied. 'You see, it was the spirit in which she brought the recommendation to the team. She was not arrogant in her approach. She simply communicated the idea in a way that supported a business case for the change. She was well aware that she had only been there for three months, and her tone and approach was deferential to the other team members.'

Bob Bee tapped his pencil on his pad. He said, 'So self-awareness plus self-motivation leads to independence?'

'I will add one more,' Dar Bee said. 'I ran into Free Bee some time after I had left that hive and asked how she was. She was good at the time, but she said that she had gone through a period in which she was feeling overwhelmed, on the verge of a burnout.'

'What had happened?' Bob Bee asked with concern.

'She had not yet attained the third aspect of successful independence.'

Dar Bee waited silently for Bob Bee to look up from his notebook and then said, 'Self-monitoring.'

'Self-monitoring?'

'Yes. The bees who have long-term success with independence must learn to channel their energies. They are often creative bees. Without the benefit of creating some boundaries, their energy and talents can become diluted.'

'What are these boundaries you speak of?'

'For example, Free Bee told me that after a few of her ideas turned into successful outcomes, bees in the organization began calling on her to help with a number of different issues or opportunities. She soon found that her own work, what she was hired to do, was not getting done. Luckily, she recognized it and created some boundaries. She created deadlines and milestones for projects she was working on. She asked her supervisor to meet with her monthly to review her work and ensure that she wasn't becoming too distracted from her core work. She knew she was talented. She did not, of course, say this part to me but it was evident. She also knew that how the other bees perceived her was important. She had a close bee buddy, and she asked her buddy to keep a check on her behaviour. Free Bee told me that she asked her buddy to let her know immediately if she was coming across as demeaning, critical, patronizing or displaying any other negative behaviour that might push the other bees away.'

'Genius!' Bob Bee expostulated.

Dar Bee said thoughtfully, 'I am describing these traits—the self-awareness, the self-motivation and the self-monitoring—as if they are distinct levels, a ladder if you will, that you build on to achieve success at being an independent bee. And in some sense, there is a certain logic to that?'

Dar Bee said the last sentence as if it were a question and then paused. Bob Bee urged her on encouragingly.

'Well, you can see as in Free Bee's case, the lines of demarcation between these levels are blurry. It is not always clear where one stops and another begins, is it?'

Bob Bee weighed Dar Bee's comments for a few moments. Then, he wrote a few more lines in his notebook and closed it. 'Dar Bee,' he said with an air of pride, 'When we try to explain something, we naturally break it down into its components, analyse it and put it back together again. We name it, codify it, convert it into terms that make sense, put it into some and sequence that makes sense to us and then we test it. You have done a wonderful job of representing why "Bee Independent" should be one of the Bee Attitudes. Consider it in!'

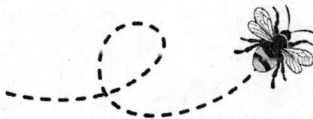

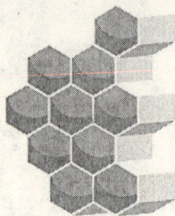

Bee Enthusiastic

Bee Attitude #14

'Pleasure in the job puts perfection in the work.'

—ARISTOTLE

'Spark Bee is always so positive,' Dar Bee said to Bob Bee.

The bees were on a very short break and Spark Bee was hovering with a small group of bees who were laughing as Bob Bee and Dar Bee passed by.

'He is next on the list,' Bob Bee said.

'Spark Bee is on your Bee Attitudes list?' Dar Bee asked doubtfully.

'Well,' corrected Bob Bee, 'Not Spark Bee himself but what he represents.'

Bob Bee let some time pass until Dar Bee couldn't stand it anymore. 'And what he represents is?' she asked playfully.

'Enthusiasm. That is what he exudes—enthusiasm!'

'So, "Bee Enthusiastic" is the next Bee Attitude?' Dar Bee inquired.

'It is. And one may ask how does a bee remain enthusiastic during times such as these, during a honey recession if you will?' he said, eyeing Dar Bee.

She took the bait and said, 'Bob Bee, I was just wondering how *does* a bee remain enthusiastic in times such as these?'

Bob Bee smiled and said, 'One chooses to be enthusiastic.'

'Chooses?'

'That's right. We actually get to choose our attitude. It's easy to be cheery and enthusiastic when things are going well. But when the challenges come, when the going gets tough, when the stressors intensify, that is when it becomes more difficult to keep the positive attitude flowing.'

Dar Bee nodded her head in agreement. 'That certainly speaks to me,' she said thoughtfully. 'When things in my life seem out of control, I recognize that my mood dampens. I feel like when I get hit with a stressful situation, I flip from a glass-half-full bee to a glass-half-empty bee.' She paused, then said, 'I don't think I have ever really thought about it being a choice though. I think I have viewed it more as a reaction or a consequence to a situation.'

'I think that is true of a lot of bees,' Bob Bee chimed in. 'I have spent some time with Spark Bee and other bees like him. There is more to these bees than what we see on the surface,' he offered.

'Such as?'

'Well, what we often see with these bees is the jovial persona that they exhibit, the cheerleader bee if you will. But this impression we get is a product of a number of characteristics that are not necessarily as visible to us.'

'I should get my diary,' Dar Bee said.

'No need,' Bob Bee replied.

Surprising Dar Bee, he said, 'I will provide the notes for you soon.' Bob Bee continued, 'These bees make a conscious choice of their attitude.'

'Got it,' Dar Bee said and saluted him jokingly. Bob Bee then listed the characteristics.

'Characteristic number one. Enthusiastic bees choose to communicate positively. I know we have already talked about communication as a Bee Attitude and you will certainly, by now, see that some of the characteristics of these Bee Attitudes overlap. Well, all those things we discussed when we talked about being a good communicator apply here. The emphasis here is on a consistent spirit of positivity.'

'Consistent spirit of positivity, eh?' Dar Bee said, looking into the distance. 'That's the hard part isn't it, the consistency?'

'It certainly is,' Bob Bee replied. 'And that is where the choice comes in. I know for a fact that Spark Bee has some intense challenges in his home, challenges that could bring any bee down. But does he bring those issues to the workplace?'

'No!' exclaimed Dar Bee.

'Actually, he does,' Bob Bee said, surprising Dar Bee again. 'Nowadays, it is extremely difficult to not let the home hive carry over into the work hive and vice versa. But Spark Bee, he talks about the challenges as opportunities and in a very inspiring light. It would be easy for him to come and complain about his burden at the home hive. For that matter, it would be easy for him to go home and complain about the stress here as well.'

Bob Bee smiled and seemed to want a response from Dar Bee.

'But he chooses to communicate positively,' she said after a few moments.

'Exactly! Now, characteristic number two. Recognizing that different bees have different perspectives.'

He saw Dar Bee's wings flutter with excitement and predicting what she wanted to say, he said, 'You might wonder what does seeing other bees' perspective have to do with enthusiasm?'

'I might,' Dar Bee replied with raised eyebrows.

'An enthusiastic bee, you see, is not just passionate about his own thoughts, ideas and framework of understanding. He wants to be, and also inspires other bees to be, enthusiastic about theirs. Spark Bee knows he can't always have the right answers to a problem. He welcomes different perspectives and ideas and weighs them against his own. When he does that, he engages the other bees. They realize that he respects their opinions and ideas even if he doesn't agree with them.'

'And thus, the name Spark Bee,' Dar Bee said coyly.

'Yes.'

'And characteristic number three?'

'Celebration of successes!' he replied.

'Partyyyy!' replied Dar Bee doing a full circle buzz.

'Something like that,' Bob Bee said looking over his spectacles. 'The enthusiastic bee understands that it is important to celebrate not only the major milestones that are successfully reached but also the smaller ones. And not just for himself. For example, Spark Bee knew that one of his fellow bee was struggling with one of his work techniques. In fact, the whole department knew. Spark Bee enlisted Rig Bee's assistance and within just a few days, the struggling bee had a perfect production day.'

'Teamwork,' Dar Bee said in a matter-of-fact manner.

'It was. But Spark Bee didn't stop there. The next day he orchestrated a short celebration event for the bee. It wasn't much. Some honey treats and a home-made medal with the words "Excellent Work" inscribed on it. The whole department took ten minutes to recognize the bee's achievement and then went back to work. It was a small effort for most of the bees in the department, but it meant everything to that one bee.'

'We really do not do enough of that type of celebrating,' Dar Bee admitted.

Bob Bee chuckled and said, 'There used to be a manager here a long time ago. Let's see, what was his nickname? Oh yeah, behind his back his department called him Miser Bee. He was a stickler for productivity.'

'I have worked with those types before.'

'That ten minutes celebration that Spark Bee arranged?'

'Yes.'

'Miser Bee would have pulled out his clip board. I can hear him mumbling even now.' Bob Bee picked up a book pretending it was a clip board and imitated Miser Bee mockingly, 'Let's see. Ten minutes. No let's make it fifteen by the time they actually get back to the work they were supposed to be doing, and...' Bob Bee then pretended to turn some pages, '...they have two hundred and twenty bees in the department.'

Bob Bee then pretended to be punching in numbers on a calculator. 'Two hundred and twenty times fifteen. Let's see, that's thirty-three hundred minutes. Thirty-three hundred minutes divided by sixty. Let's see. That's fifty-five bee-hours wasted all because they decided to celebrate because some bee did what he was actually supposed to do the day before.' Bob Bee threw his mock clip board on the table and exclaimed, 'Report! They are all going on report!'

Dar Bee could barely contain herself laughing. 'Yes,' she sputtered. 'I certainly know the type.'

Bob Bee regained his composure and stated, 'What those bees like Miser Bee do not understand is that those meagre ten minutes is an investment and will lead to better productivity. They were celebrating the fact that a bee who was struggling made it through the struggle and attained a high level of competency in a skill that benefits the hive. Do you think that bee knows with certainty what the department's priorities are? Do you think that bee now knows the level of support he has? Do you think that bee is more likely to stay when the challenges of productivity go up?'

'Off your soap box,' Dar Bee said with a smile. 'Yes, yes and yes. We are on the same page here.'

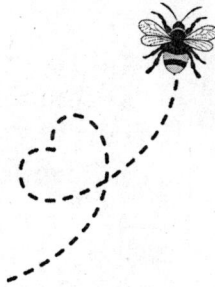

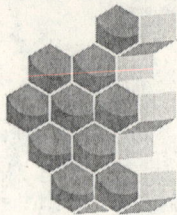

The Unveiling of the Last Bee Attitude

Bee Attitude #15

*'A mind that is stretched by new experience
can never go back to its old dimensions.'*

—OLIVER WENDELL HOLMES, JR

Spring and summer passed. The bees of the hive did, in fact, produce enough honey to comfortably survive the coming winter. At Bob Bee's recommendation, Queen Bee approved a celebration for the hard work the bees had put in.

'How did you get her to go for that?' Dar Bee asked Bob Bee after she had found out about the upcoming event.

'The Queen Bee?' he responded. 'Oh, she's not heartless you know. She knows that the bees worked hard.'

'And she got what she wanted,' Dar Bee put in with a slight air of sarcasm.

Bob Bee considered his response. Finally, he said, 'Queen Bee deals with challenges and issues that the rest of the hive has no idea about.' He could see that his initial response had surprised Dar Bee. 'Trust me,' he continued, 'I have my own issues with her. There are many things I would do differently from her. But I am trying to give her the benefit of the doubt.'

'You are a very kind bee,' Dar Bee said genuinely.

'Well, I am not so sure about that,' he said with mock embarrassment. 'But I do try to remind myself daily that we all have different roles and different perspectives. What's the saying? Fly a mile in another bee's wings before you judge her?'

They both laughed. 'So, this celebration. What's the plan? What's the venue?' Dar Bee asked.

'It is in two weeks,' Bob Bee replied. 'There will be food and music and...' he gave a dramatic pause to draw Dar Bee in.

'And?' she finally said.

'And a big surprise.'

'Do tell!' Dar Bee said with intrigue.

'Can't.'

'Can't or won't?' Dar Bee said, a bit dismayed.

'Both,' Bob Bee replied wryly.

'Now that is not fair,' Dar Bee complained. 'I have been right by your side through this whole thing. Surely, you could give a little insight to your good friend Dar Bee,' she urged.

'You make a good point,' Bob Bee replied. 'How about I give you a bit of a hint?'

'If that is all you are willing to give, I will take it,' she said in a disappointed tone.

'Well, you know that so far we have fourteen Bee Attitudes?'

Dar Bee, who had not been counting the Bee Attitudes, pulled out her diary. It took her a few minutes, but she finally looked up and said, 'That's correct, fourteen.'

Dar Bee could tell Bob Bee was excited. 'There is actually one more Bee Attitude on my list that we haven't discussed.'

'Really!' Dar Bee said. She was very surprised. 'What is it?' she asked eagerly.

'Well, that is the surprise, isn't it?'

'You mean...?'

Bob Bee stopped her with a wing up. 'You are a good friend, Dar Bee. I really am not trying to be coy here. There is some work to be done to appropriately introduce this Bee Attitude. I have told you more than I am planning to tell anyone else. I am asking you to trust me on this.'

Dar Bee sighed. 'All right,' she said in defeat. 'But...'

Again, Bob Bee interjected, 'You will have a front row seat. I promise.'

The next two weeks were busy for Dar Bee, as she was in charge of doing inventory. She remained interested in what Bob Bee was doing to prepare for the celebration but did not have time to ask many questions.

Bob Bee was also busy preparing for the celebration. There were rumours of a photographer being hired and bees being asked to have their pictures taken. These rumours were, in fact, true. However, Bob Bee, who had arranged for the photographers, got each bee being photographed to sign a nondisclosure agreement. There was talk that the celebration was being catered and that there would be special honey with exotic spices in them. There were also rumours that the famous band, The Bees' Knees, was slated to do the entertainment. Bob Bee would not comment on this. By the time the day of celebration came, the colony was truly buzzing.

A large turnout was expected, so some modifications had been made to the hive to accommodate all the bees in one space. The food was placed in an adjacent room and there were several bees with chef's hats on ready to serve. There were signs coming into the hall that read, 'Well Done', 'Excellent Work', 'Teamwork' and, of course, 'To Bee or Not To Bee'. The doors were opened, and the bees flew in.

The first thing the bees noticed was a makeshift stage at the far end of the room with some hover chairs in place. Above the stage, covering most of the wall, was a thin, rectangular object covered by a sheet. There was much buzzing and speculation about what was behind the sheet. The shape connoted that it was likely a framed picture. The bees whispered to one another and many bet it was a picture of Queen Bee with her slogan 'To Bee or Not To Bee' over her head.

The bees rotated in and out of the auditorium and the adjacent room, with the eating and buzzing. After some time, there was some music as well. The bees looked to the stage and somehow The Bees' Knees had slipped on stage and had begun playing their latest hit single, 'Honey, You Are the Only Bee for Me'. The bees began hovering to and fro to the music. After the song, the lead bee said, 'Don't go away. I think there are a few awards to give out and then we will be back.' The crowd cheered.

The band left the stage and a couple of bees brought a podium out. The crowd went silent and in hovered Queen Bee to the podium.

'Well, that was a buzz kill,' one bee whispered a little too loudly to the bee next to him.

'Shh!' the other bee whispered back in embarrassment.

Queen Bee tapped the microphone with her wing to confirm that the sound system was working. 'I will not be up here for long,' she began. The bee who had whispered about her being a buzz kill could have sworn she was looking directly at him. 'Some months ago,' she continued with her queenly voice, 'I hovered in front of you and presented a challenge. It was a challenge to each of you and to the colony as a whole. We were facing a potential honey recession because of factors outside our control. I asked you to fly further and work harder, so we could meet the production quotas to get us through the winter. I asked you to consider if you were to bee or not to bee.' She paused and scanned the crowd slowly.

To the audience's surprise, Queen Bee pulled a tissue from a recess in the podium and began wiping tears from her eyes. After a few moments, she blew her nose and then cleared her voice with a cough. Regaining her composure, she said, 'I am proud of every bee in this room. You buzzed up and did what you needed to do through a very stressful period.'

Giving a nod to Bob Bee who was hovering off to the side of the stage, she added with a smile, 'And with guidance from our honourable Bee Resource Director, you did it without killing each other.' Queen Bee hovered backed from the podium, faced Bob Bee, and began clapping her wings. Immediately, the crowd joined her in earnest. Bob Bee blushed.

Queen Bee returned to the podium and the cheers finally subsided. 'I want you to know that I am sincerely grateful to be a part of this beehive and I thank you from the bottom of my heart for what you do and what you mean to me.'

Those who were in front of the crowd noticed that she squelched another round of tears. She looked back at the bee who made that 'buzz kill' comment and smiled. 'I promised I would not be up here long. Bob Bee has some very important awards to give so please celebrate with him and those who receive these awards. And don't forget to celebrate your own accomplishments.'

With that, Queen Bee slowly flew out of the room.

Bob Bee hovered to the stage. He began by saying, 'I hope all of you are enjoying the celebration so far.'

The crowd cheered.

Holding both wings up to stop the cheering, he finally said, 'We will have The Bees' Knees back on stage soon.'

More cheering.

Over his glasses, he peered at Dar Bee, who indeed had a front row seat. After the cheering subsided, he said, 'This is a very important year for me in many ways.' The room was silent. 'I will be retiring this year,' he went on to say.

He saw Dar Bee move uncomfortably in her chair. Through the rumble of the crowd, a few discernible words made it to his ears. 'You can't retire', 'please stay', 'you are the best bee resource director' and 'we love you, Bob Bee'.

Again, he put his wings up and waited for the rumblings to cease. 'For a few people, including myself, I needed to get that message out there.' Before the rumblings could resume, he said quickly, 'But today is not about me. It is about recognizing some extraordinary bees. These bees have helped shape who we are as a colony and many of these bees have played extremely important roles in getting us through this recession.'

Again, the crowd cheered.

'I will ask for your patience,' Bob Bee said from behind the podium. 'We will honour fifteen bees and I plan to say a few words about each of them. Each of them, in their own way, have made sacrifices, so I am hoping that a small portion of your day to honour them will not inconvenience you.' The response that he gauged from the crowd was positive.

'We have set up the stage and when I call out the bee's name, I will ask him or her to come up on stage and take a seat facing the audience. I was given the honour of naming these awards and I want to give you a little background on that. I am calling the awards the Bee Attitudes.' Some bees smiled and other bees looked at one another with confusion.

'They are,' Bob Bee continued, 'a list of traits or characteristics that are conducive to building a better bee and a stronger organization. These are tangible traits; that is, other bees can see the actionable things these bees do for that betterment. I call them the Bee Attitudes because I believe our actions are largely guided by our attitudes.'

He paused and there was mild clapping from the audience. 'I am confident you will understand this more deeply as we give out the awards.'

Looking over at the front row, he said, 'Dar Bee, would you mind assisting me with the awards?'

Dar Bee was fairly sure her cheeks had turned pink by the warm glow she felt in them. 'I would be more than happy to,' she replied after only a short hesitation.

Surprising Dar Bee, Bob Bee said to the audience, 'It will not be a surprise to many of you that Dar Bee has been assisting me with much of the bee resource needs during this crisis. You have seen us side by side over the past months working together to do what we can to help. She has been very insightful and instrumental in guiding many of us through some of the day-to-day struggles we have seen with this recession, and I think it only fitting that she be a part of this ceremony.'

If her cheeks were pink before, they were scarlet now. She squeaked out a 'thank you' and hovered to Bob Bee's side. Bob Bee took a covering off a rather large table in the room. The crowd saw fifteen trophies glistening there. Bob Bee hovered back to the microphone. He said, 'What I would like to do is provide a description of each bee and his or her characteristics and contribution that culminates in announcing his or her name.'

The crowd assented.

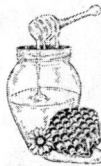

Award #1: Bee Knowledgeable

'All right. Let's get started then. The first Bee Attitude award…' There was a drum roll from The Bees' Knees drummer who had perhaps had a little too much honey and had been quietly hovering behind the drums. Bob Bee resumed, 'The first Bee Attitude award goes to a bee that stays busy all the time. This bee recently learnt that speed to production is not a substitute for quality. She learnt that it was very important for her to be knowledgeable about her roles and that sometimes even subtle changes in the process can produce unwarranted results.'

Noticing that the audience had become silent, Bob Bee said, 'Now, you may be wondering why I am mentioning what this bee was doing wrong. You may be thinking I thought this was an awards ceremony, a ceremony to honour success.'

He peered over his glasses and slowly scanned the audience. He asked in an authoritative voice, 'Who among us has not spilled some precious nectar?' He allowed the question to sink in. 'We are here to celebrate successes. You will hear today of bees who have had longstanding successes and also about bees who, during this critical time for our colony, were shown or actually showed us how to improve. Their awareness of the opportunity, them embracing the attitude to be better and their decision to act on the opportunity, well that does not show weakness, my friends. That demonstrates strength!'

Bob Bee could see heads nodding affirmatively and he felt like he had gotten his message across. 'So then, this bee listened to the advice that was provided and even asked for more. We noticed over the course of this critical period that she sought out educational opportunities to improve her skills and found mentors who were willing to help. This bee exemplifies the criteria of the first Bee Attitude which is to 'Bee Knowledgeable'. Lady bees and gentlebees, please clap your wings together for our own Busy Bee!'

The crowd cheered and hovered side to side as Busy Bee made her way to the stage. Dar Bee handed her the 'Bee Knowledgeable' trophy and escorted her to her hover seat. Busy Bee was blushing as she waved to the audience.

Award #2: Bee Dependable

Bob Bee then moved on to the next award.

'The next award on the list hits close to home for me. After a conversation with this bee, I realized I needed to tell our supervisors that we had done a poor job of communicating our expectations. I realized we must improve on that. But we were falling short on production. So, I posed to this bee that the worker bees should ask how they can become more dependable. I asked if they could count on each other? Could management count on them? I assured this bee that the worker bees could count on management in the future. We discussed that dependability goes both ways. Will we show up on time? Will we stay focussed to ensure our part of the work is completed accurately and on time? Will we step up and help our fellow bee when we see them lagging? Will we ask for help when we are having difficulties?'

Bob Bee took a quick pause. The audience, he believed, was listening intently. 'Don't get me wrong. This bee asked his fair share of questions too. When we were done, we both did what we said we were going to do. We received feedback from our respective constituents and then we took action.' Another pause. 'The production stayed above expectations since then. Lady bees and gentlebees, please join me in congratulating our own May Bee!'

Like Busy Bee, May Bee hovered his way through the crowd and accepted the trophy from Dar Bee in front of a cheering audience.

Award #3: Bee Flexible

After the cheers subsided and May Bee was seated, Bob Bee continued, 'Our next honouree helped us all understand that it is okay to ask questions when faced with a change. In fact, it is more than okay. Management has a high degree of respect for those workers who ask questions in a respectful manner. It challenges our current process and makes us a better organization. As you can see, our colony has to adapt to the changing external pressures. Those bees who want to make themselves indispensable understand that they have to adapt as well. This recipient has demonstrated true flexibility in this critical time of our colony and has won the 'Bee Flexible' award. Give it up for our own But Bee.'

The pattern of Dar Bee awarding the trophy and the crowd cheering continued.

Award #4: Bee Innovative

Bob Bee knew that he had several more awards to give out and soon the crowd would be anxious for the band to return. He decided to accelerate the pace.

'Our next bee was the impetus for a six per cent increase in production during this stressful period. Her innovative spirit guided the team in reducing waste, reducing down-time and ensuring the activities of the bees in her department added value to the outcome, the honey. We need bees who think outside the hive, who bring their ideas to help us be better. Our 'Bee Innovative' award goes to the one and only Rig Bee!'

Award #5: Bee Authentic

'Bogus Bee, come on up!' Bob Bee belted out after the cheers for Rig Bee died down. As Bogus Bee hovered to the stage, Bob Bee announced, 'This Bee has learnt that he needs to be true to himself, and that he has skills that can add value to the organization. Management learnt that we have the responsibility of matching those skills to the right part of the colony. His change in behaviour has given a number of bees the freedom to openly discuss their skill sets with their supervisors and find a better fit. Congratulations, Bogus Bee.'

Award #6: Bee a Great Communicator

'Communication is the exchange of accurate meaning between two or more bees,' Bob Bee said before announcing the next award winner. 'And no bee has come farther in this category than our own Gab Bee.' He motioned her to the stage. 'When she realized how some of her communication was affecting her co-workers, she made a change and began focussing on positive messaging and active listening.'

Gab Bee's department cheered the loudest.

Award #7: Bee Curious

'I was informed just before the ceremony that the next winner is first cousins with Rig Bee,' Bob Bee resumed at the podium. 'He is called Sweat Bee because he asks so many questions that his supervisor once said it made him sweat.'

The crowd, who knew Sweat Bee, laughed. As Sweat

Bee made his way to the stage, Bob Bee said, 'Thank you for giving us the motivation to ask what and when and why and how and where in the spirit of improving our work. Thank you for being curious.'

Award #8: Bee Frank

Bob Bee continued to the next award, saying, 'There will be some of you who haven't met our next award winner. He agreed to come out of retirement and assist us in an area that we needed help with. And that area is the need to be open and honest with one another; that is, not watering down our opinions, ideas and suggestions but making sure that they are conveyed in a spirit of respectfulness. Please join me in honouring the one and only Frank Bee!'

Award #9: Bee Kind

Again, after the cheers died out, Bob Bee said in his best announcer voice, 'Phil Bee come on up!' As Phil Bee made his way to the stage, Bob Bee said, 'Phil Bee has gone above and beyond to infuse kindness into the way he approaches his colleagues. You, no doubt by now, have seen some of the overlap in some of the characteristics of the recipients of these awards. We have intentionally called each of these individual awards out because we believe they deserve attention.'

As Dar Bee handed Phil Bee his award, Bob Bee said, 'Kindness needs to be integrated into the way we approach one another all the time.'

Award #10: Bee Humble

As expected, Humble Bee blushed when her name was called. Her peers had to urge her up to the stage. 'Do all of you know Humble Bee?' Bob Bee asked loudly. The crowd went wild. After Humble Bee was seated, Bob Bee simply said, 'Thank you so much for what you have quietly done during this stressful time. Your unassuming manner has been particularly helpful to many of the New Bees. Humility trumps arrogance every time.'

Award #11: Bee Ambitious

Dar Bee knew that 'Bee Ambitious' was the next award. She also knew that throughout her discussions with Bob Bee, they had not identified a particular bee with this trait. She wondered who the winner was. Bob Bee looked to the audience and asked rhetorically, 'Who do you know who competes against herself to become better at her job. Her motives are selfless. She is not practising any one-upbeeship with her team. Who do you know who is eager to learn? Who is very self-aware.'

The audience murmured among themselves, and Bob Bee allowed just enough time before he continued. 'She has demonstrated leadership in this characteristic over and over the years. The 'Bee Ambitious' award goes to…'

To Dar Bee's surprise, Bob Bee turned to face her and the current award winners and said, '…Our very own Dar Bee!'

Apparently, Bob Bee had pre-arranged this particular award with Phil Bee who hovered up and handed Dar Bee her award. She cried as the crowd erupted again in applause.

Award #12: Bee a Team Player

With this, Bob Bee moved on to the next award, saying, 'Next, we have a bee that believes our Queen, our drones, our worker bees, all our different bees have different roles, but he does not believe one is better or more important than the other. His behaviour demonstrates that the sum of our skills as a team is greater than the individual parts. The "Bee a Team Player" award goes out to Lowell Bee.'

Lowell Bee brought his entire team up to the stage with him, but they quickly realized there wasn't enough room for all of them to accommodate all of them.

Award #13: Bee Independent

'The next award,' Bob Bee resumed after all of Lowell Bee's team members left the stage, 'reflects a high level of self-awareness, a high level of self-motivation and a high level of self-monitoring.' At this point, he could tell he was losing the audience. 'In short,' he added, 'This bee is an independent thinker. Now that may surprise some of you since the last award was for being a team player.' He turned and smiled at Dar Bee. 'We want individual bees to optimize their ideas and talents. So, while we will continue to operate with a high level of teamwork, we encourage this type of independence. While there are many deserving candidates from within our own hive, we thought we should think outside the hive for this one, and award this to the bee who inspired this trait to be added in the Bee Attitudes list. The Bee Attitude Award to "Bee Independent" goes to Dar Bee's former colleague from another hive, Free Bee.'

Award #14: Bee Enthusiastic

'We need bees who bring energy to our work, bees who communicate positively, bees who recognize and respect that other bees have different perspectives, bees that inspire other bees and bees who know how to celebrate successes,' Bob Bee stated with authority. The audience knew exactly who the next winner was. 'The one. The only. Here he is...Spark Bee.'

Spark Bee made his way to the stage with a noise maker in his mouth and coloured streamers trailing behind him. The audience's cheer was now the highest it had been for the entire celebration.

Award #15: The Unveiling of the Last Bee Attitude

It took several minutes to silence the crowd. Bob Bee said, 'Thank you for your patience and your participation in these awards. I only have one more award to present and then we will resume the celebrations.'

The Bees' Knees moved to the side of the stage. Bob Bee gestured to some bees who were now hovering by whatever was behind the sheet on the wall. He nodded and the bees adjusted some ropes that caused the top of the structure to move forward by a few inches. Bob Bee asked the award winners to turn and look at the structure. They did so.

'This next award is complicated,' Bob Bee began. 'The criteria are complex and so it is difficult to achieve.' He nodded to the hovering bees and, in tandem, they released the ropes and the sheet fell to the ground gracefully. The room fell silent. In a beautiful, gold frame was a picture, containing the faces of everyone who had received an award, in a collage style. Dar Bee noticed her picture was different than the others and surmised that Bob Bee had had the photographer take her picture surreptitiously.

Bob Bee judged that a sufficient amount of time had passed, and with his deepest and sincerest voice, he said, 'What you are looking at is a picture of Commitment.' He allowed the words to sink in. 'All of these bees that you see, all that they represent, you see, that is commitment. It is something each of us—me, management, Queen Bee, worker bees—all of us, should strive for each day.'

With a final nod to the hovering bees, they worked together and pulled the previously unnoticed gold tape from the top and bottom of the frame. When they were done, the top of the frame read 'TO BEE OR NOT TO BEE' and the bottom of the frame read 'BEE COMMITTED'.

'So,' Bob Bee said, 'This year, the "Bee Committed" award goes to all of you on the stage.' He turned to the crowd and ended with, 'I know each one of you is worthy of an award for getting us through this recession. I salute you and wish you the best in the coming year.'

He gestured to the band who made their way to the stage while the crowd applauded, whistled and cheered.

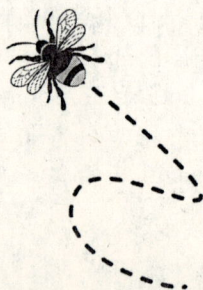

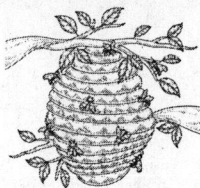

Building a 'Better Buzz'

Dar Bee had not been able to talk to Bob Bee after the ceremony and was disappointed. However, she was pleased to see a note on her desk the next morning asking her to join Bob Bee for breakfast.

'Come in! Come in,' Bob Bee said, waving her in. On his desk a nice breakfast was laid out.

'I can't believe you are retiring,' Dar Bee said mournfully. 'Why didn't you tell me?'

'I just didn't think the time was right,' he replied. 'We needed to get through this recession, and I did not want to distract you.'

He gestured to a wrapped package on the desk.

'For me?' she asked. 'What's the occasion?'

'I am formally passing my list of Bee Attitudes on to you. I am confident you will know what to do with them,' Bob Bee said proudly.

She opened the package and began thumbing through the Bee Attitudes. Bob Bee sipped his honey. After a few minutes, she said, 'Oh my. There is a lot more in here than what we have talked about.'

Dar Bee thought she saw Bob Bee become a bit misty-eyed. He said, 'I consider that to be my life's work.' He regained his composure and added, 'When you have time to read through this more thoroughly, you will certainly find some of your findings and recommendations that you have communicated to me in there as well.'

'I don't know how to thank you,' Dar Bee said, wiping a tear escaping from her eyes.

'Well,' Bob Bee said in his authoritative voice, 'I do.'

This surprised Dar Bee.

'You can thank me by accepting the position of bee resource director.'

Her mouth gaped open.

'Already cleared it with Queen Bee and the committee,' Bob Bee said. 'All you have to do is say yes and you start on Monday.'

Dar Bee hugged Bob Bee. Then, she held the Bee Attitudes book next to her heart and said, 'Yes. Of course, I will accept the position. You can count on me to be a good steward of these Bee Attitudes.'

And with that, she carried them out to the colony.

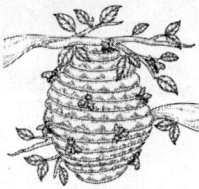

Bee Attitudes: The Book

The first time Dar Bee opened the Bee Attitudes book after Bob Bee retired, she found that he had left her a note:

Dear Dar Bee,

I trust you are doing well. You will remember that I mentioned a couple of times that the characteristics of these Bee Attitudes can overlap. I believe it is worthwhile to look at each one deeply and then pull back to look at the entire list. You will note that each Bee Attitude has suggested action items. These action items have been accumulated over time. It is not necessary that each action applies to all bees. Instead, each bee should evaluate the suggested action relative to where they are in their own journey. To that end, I have tried to provide working definitions of each to level-set our understanding, so that we are all buzzing off the same sheet of music. At the end of these Bee Attitudes, I have provided two surveys. The first is a self-perception survey that encourages each bee to rate him or herself on a scale of 1 (Poor) to 10 (Excellent) in each Bee Attitude. This may be helpful in identifying what areas the bee should consider working on first. The second survey is a little riskier and must be handled with care. In this survey, which is the same as the first, another bee will rate how they perceive the bee is doing on the same scale. You will see the importance of handling this one with anonymity. I know you will be a wonderful steward of these Bee Attitudes.

All my best,
Bob Bee

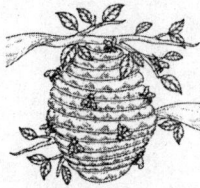

Bee Attitude Action Items

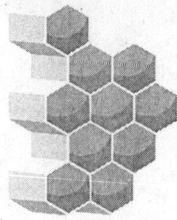

Bee Attitude #1

Bee Knowledgeable

Have a thorough understanding of your job. Know the principles, the tasks and the intricacy of how doing your job correctly affects the entire work process, the other team members and the end product or service.

Follow the action items given below diligently to follow through on this Bee Attitude:

- Ask questions with the desire to learn and improve.
- View less than optimal outcomes as an opportunity to learn (even if it is learning what not to do next time).
- Find a mentor who knows the business and put on your 'listening ears'.
- Take orientation seriously. Ingest all the information you can.
- If there is a policy, know the policy.
- If there is a procedure, know the procedure.
- Learn your role inside and out.
- Get certified in your area of expertise.
- When you are new to a position, listen more than you talk.
- Make sure expectations are clear.
- Find networking opportunities that will help you enhance your knowledge base and skills.

- Join expert groups or associations.
- Create a professional development plan.
- Read, read and read.
- Set goals for your development. Small goals today are stepping stones for future success.
- Gain clarity on what you need to accomplish.
- Embrace the learning process. Ask questions, be inquisitive and embrace curiosity.
- Volunteer to teach others. When you put yourself in a position to teach, it will cause you to deepen your commitment to and understanding of the subject.
- Volunteer to be a speaker on a topic that will push you out of your comfort zone.
- Volunteer to be a go-to expert for someone with less experience.
- Connect with others who have more experience than you.
- Shadow experts to learn best practices.
- Talk to peers working in other offices and companies, and learn from them.
- Look for ways to improve processes.
- Say yes to new opportunities and experiences.
- Take action. Learn for growth. Don't let fear freeze you.
- Know what attitude you choose. You have a choice to be positive or negative, be open to new ideas or be cynical, show kindness or be critical of others, be genuinely helpful or show self-serving behaviours, etc.
- Focus on the choices you make at the beginning of your day.
- Ask valuable questions to your seniors and peers

such as, 'Knowing what you know now, what advice would you give someone in my role?' or 'What do you wish you had done differently when you were in my current role?'

- After taking on a new project or responsibility, ask for direct feedback of what you did well and what you could have done better.

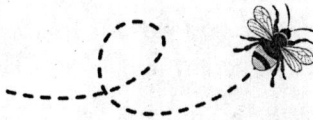

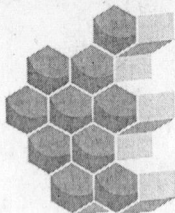

Bee Attitude #2

Bee Dependable

Be the individual that your co-workers, family and friends can consistently count on.

Follow the action items given below diligently to follow through on this Bee Attitude:

- Be prepared for meetings. Ask for the agenda and objectives of the meeting in advance if not provided.
- Arrive to meetings on time. Actually, arrive early and stay focussed in meetings.
- Recognize that everyone has a responsibility to contribute to the success of meetings. This is different than just showing up as a warm body. Be engaged and share your ideas.
- Know your productivity expectations and where you are in reference to them.
- If you see that you cannot do what you have committed to, inform the right people as timely as possible. Ask for help and guidance.
- Own your mistakes.
- Recognize when others are struggling and offer help to them.
- Understand what your quality product or service looks like and keep that as a priority in your mind.

- Focus on the results, not just the activities.
- Know what is expected of you and the timeline for completion up front.
- Ask questions if you are uncertain about expectations.
- Be clear on your role. Are you the one completing the work, part of a team, the go-to lead or the formal or informal leader of the team?
- Remember, consistency creates your personal reputation.
- Identify the impression you want others to have of you, and then create it.
- Become a dependable team member. Help others learn and grow, and provide encouragement.
- Become the go-to person for feedback and reflection.
- Listen with the intention of really understanding and learning.
- Make sure your behaviours match your words.
- Evaluate your dependability behaviours. If there are recurring circumstances in which you have not proven to be dependable, it is time to make a positive change.
- Remember, people evaluate your dependability based on your actions, not your intentions. Actions speak louder than words (and thoughts)!
- Dependability also shows up in communication. Ask yourself if people count on you to be honest and truthful with them, even if it isn't always positive. Be willing to share valuable feedback that will help someone learn and grow. Be the one they count on for meaningful feedback.

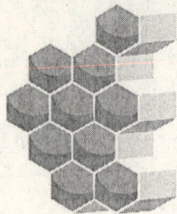

Bee Attitude #3

Bee Flexible

Recognize that the market for products and services change, processes change, technology changes. Recognize that relationships evolve. Greet these changes with enthusiasm and a spirit of seeking progress. Do not be the 'that's the way we've always done it' person.

Follow the action items given below diligently to follow through on this Bee Attitude:

- Recognize that 'my way or the highway' is usually the wrong way.
- Keep an open mind towards new ideas.
- Cross-train when you can.
- When you see a problem, look for a solution instead of complaining.
- Develop your skill sets. This will allow you to stretch.
- Set stretch goals and challenge yourself.
- Listen to the voice inside your head. Ask yourself what your immediate response to a change is. If you feel reluctant to a change, ask questions in the right spirit to learn the reasons behind the change.
- Determine if you welcome new ideas and look for new possibilities, or stand firm to keep things the way they are now.

- Recognize that in the ever-changing work environment, flexibility is a powerful skill for success.
- Learn with purpose. Recognize that what is new to you today will be your expertise in the future.
- Make learning fun. Play games that involve teaching others about new processes.
- Listen, listen, listen. If you are always talking, it is hard to learn and be flexible.
- Just like physical stretching, use mindfulness to embrace new ideas. Exercise and expand your mind to new ideas, philosophies and approaches.
- Hold up a mirror to yourself and evaluate your flexibility. Ask a friend to provide feedback on your flexibility and willingness to try new ideas.
- Accept feedback as an opportunity to improve and get better.
- Don't just focus on your intention (what you hope to do), but look at your impact (what you actually did). Look for alignment and inconsistencies between words and behaviours.
- Look for trends in the feedback from others. Determine if others comment on you being controlling—that you need to always be in charge, that you need to be the boss or that you need to do things your way.
- Feedback can be a wonderful gift if we receive it, hear it and process it. Check for yourself.

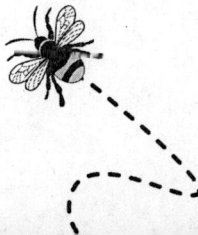

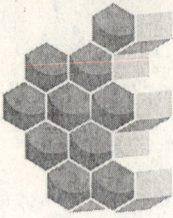

Bee Attitude #4

Bee Innovative

Think of ways to work smarter. Create an atmosphere that promotes creativity and improves efficiency, quality, outcomes, services and team dynamics. In your important personal relationships, try new experiences together.

Follow the action items given below diligently to follow through on this Bee Attitude:

- Find technology that will leverage your time.
- Don't just criticize the current process. Rather, offer constructive suggestions.
- Identify inefficiencies and potential solutions.
- Don't wait to be told to be innovative. Activate your imagination and get started!
- Embrace your work with a focus on continuous improvement.
- Seek ways to reduce steps, save time, save money, improve quality and create a better experience for your clients.
- Focus on the feeling of victory and accomplishment when innovation is activated. It can be positive, empowering and encouraging.
- Listen to the language of those around you. Determine

if your team embraces an improvement mindset and celebrates creative thinking.

- Identify someone in your organization who demonstrates an innovative mindset. Meet with this person and learn from them. Ask what drives their focus. Become a student of innovation.
- Ask 'what if' questions to activate possibility thinking.
- Ask probing questions that begin with 'how, what and where'.
- Learn something new about someone else.
- Stop multitasking. Give your full attention to what is in front of you.
- Notice the innovation in your community: new housing additions, coffee shops, restaurants, businesses, etc.
- Begin something new for your mind, body and spirit.
- Celebrate the successes of others and recognize their innovative spirit.
- Remember, failure is a part of the process. Don't let it hold you back. Embrace it!

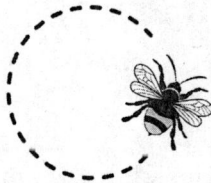

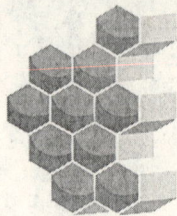

Bee Attitude #5

Bee Authentic

Do not let there be gaps between who you say you are and who you really are. Be genuine in a spirit of community. Seek out the right fit for you in your work setting.

Follow the action items given below diligently to follow through on this Bee Attitude:

- Identify your values, your beliefs and what is most important to you.
- Be clear on how your values and beliefs show up in your daily behaviours.
- Recognize when your words and actions are in conflict with your values and beliefs.
- Think in advance about how you would respond if you experienced a conflict of values (when a situation in your environment is at odds with your personal values and beliefs).
- Identify moments when you bring your authentic self and areas where you hide or mask your true feelings.
- Ask yourself what you can learn from those moments when you are your most authentic self.
- Determine the people in your life who see your most authentic self. Ask them for feedback or guidance.

- Ask yourself what you can learn from those moments when you are less authentic and identify what causes you to be less authentic with some people. Also observe what you need to be more authentic in those moments.
- Identify how you being authentic (or not authentic) impacts those around you.
- Identify how behaving as your true self impacts your confidence in self.
- Stay in touch with your values, beliefs and strengths. Know those activities that fuel you and give you energy.
- Recognize those activities that drain you and sap your energy, and avoid them when possible.
- Find opportunities where you can work in your strengths path (your authentic self) most of the time.
- Recognize the moments when vulnerability helps strengthen relationships at work and at home.
- Ask a trusted friend or colleague for feedback about your behaviours in action.
- Identify one or two areas where you would like to be more authentic.
- In moments of uncertainty, be honest and speak your truth respectfully.
- Create a gratitude journal. This can provide perspective of blessings both big and small, and help you appreciate your authentic self.

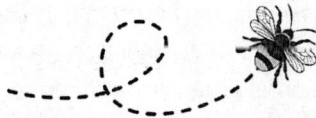

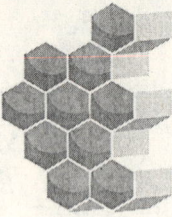

Bee Attitude #6

Bee a Great Communicator

Remember that communication is the exchange of meaning between two or more individuals. Consistently seek clarity in these exchanges. Choose the right words, tone and body language for the occasion. Assess the same in your audience as they provide feedback. Listen intently in search of understanding others.

Follow the action items given below diligently to follow through on this Bee Attitude. For this Bee Attitude we have used an A–Z format for the action items to highlight the nuances and intricacies of communication.

- *Avoid Assumptions*: We know the filters that can cause the sender and receiver to not be on the same page during a communication. Do not take for granted or consider it a foregone conclusion that those you are communicating with are on the same page as you. Be hypervigilant to maintain an awareness of these filters and make adjustments to promote clarity and consistency of communication.

- *Build Bridges*: When you practise avoiding assumptions, you begin moving towards giving others the benefit of the doubt. And then what happens to your communication? You develop a cadence of communication where you are joining and connecting in a way that adds value. Then, you are building bridges, not walls.

- *Construct Context*: There's so much that gets lost if the context around your communication is not set. And there is so much to be gained when you and the other person are clear about it. Setting context means you are creating the right space for your communication to be understood the way you intended.

- *Dispel Distractions*: There is enough competition for your full attention. It is imperative that you do all you can to remove the distractions that can be an obstacle to what is important in the communication. Turn off the devices in your hands and the scripts running in your head, and concentrate on the other person's side in the communication.

- *Express Expectations*: You expect certain things out of yourself and other people, in both your personal and work relationships. It might be productivity, completion of tasks or specific behaviours, the list goes on. How can you reduce disappointments in yourself and others, relative to these expectations? You must express them. Not in a dictatorial way, but in a way that promotes input and buy-in when others are involved. For those important things in your life, set a goal or define a target.

- *Frame Feedback*: Ken Blanchard said that 'feedback is the breakfast of champions'. You all need to give and get it. Give constructive feedback privately and praise feedback publicly. Focus on the behaviour, not the person and use your skills to build bridges.

- *Get Gender/Generation*: Men and women may

communicate differently. One is not right or the other wrong. Give the other the benefit of the doubt and work hard to find the meaning in the communication. There is much we can learn from different generations. And there is perhaps much we can teach other generations as well. There are likely to be different assumptions and different contexts. Use your focus and skills to bridge the divide and find meaning in the communication.

- *Hold 'Howevers'*: Be careful with words like 'however', 'although' and 'but' in your conversations. Use words like 'and' or 'also' to add to the conversation.

- *Inhibit Interruptions*: Be patient. Be courteous. Let the other person finish what they are saying. Not interrupting is a precursor to listening loyally.

- *Jam Judgement*: Similar to inhibiting interruption, where you need to hold on to what you want to say until the other is finished, when you jam judgement, you are mentally holding on to the decision as to where you stand, your choice of a perspective, until you have addressed the things that might skew your judgement.

- *Kindle Kindness*: Communication is about exchanging meaning, not meanness. Kindling kindness is about the spirit of the exchange. Mastering some or all of these A–Zs of communication will bring you closer to consistency in kindling kindness, but the choice to be kind in your communication is just that—a choice. A constant vigilance to be kind will elevate your communication effectiveness.

- *Listen Loyally*: One of the kindest things you can do

is listen loyally. Listen all the way to the end without writing your story in. Listen with interest. Listen with empathy. Listen without letting your mind wander. And listen with the intent to understand, rather than respond.

- *Manage Messages*: One way to show you are listening loyally and to show respect is to respond to your messages in a timely manner. When you get a text, an e-mail or some other electronic communication, give the sender a signal that you received it. You might not know the answer to what they are asking immediately but close the communication loop and don't leave the important people in your organization wondering if you received their message.

- *Nest in the Now*: Stay present in your communications. Consciously set aside the scripts running through your head and close the electronic devices. Stay focussed in the present and on the people.

- *Own Order*: Power differentials influence communication. It can be easy to find yourself being overly deferential to someone in a perceived position of power (for instance, a boss). Likewise, you may, when you are in the perceived position of power, unwittingly influence the communication in an unintended manner. Keep these power differentials in check and be careful that you do not allow them to skew the true intended messages.

- *Practise Persuasion*: You will want and need to influence others' behaviours. We are all both logical and emotional beings. With credibility as your backdrop, use data, information and stories to motivate others to change their minds, actions and behaviours. Note that the word is influence, not manipulate.

- *Query Quiet*: Silence can have multiple meanings, but do not be mistaken, for it *does* have meaning. Listen to the quiet and see what it is saying. Assess the silence in the context of the situation, the tone of the prior conversation and power differential. By reading what it means, include silence in the conversation.

- *Risk Recovery*: You will make mistakes. You will say things you wish you hadn't. You will do things you regret. When you do, something is lost or taken away in the conversation or in the relationship. Knowing when to say sorry will likely give you a chance to get back to clear communication.

- *Scrap Scoring*: Communication is not a competition. It is a platform to exchange meaning to one another. Keeping score implies a winner and a loser. You will win when you focus on ensuring the accurate exchange of information without adding stories of who was 'bigger, better, stronger or faster'.

- *Take Time*: We live in a fast-paced society. Everything is 'instant'. You must be careful that your communication responses are not *reactive*. Instead, be *responsive*. And what's the difference? The difference is the time and space between the communication stimulus and the response to it. You should, in important communications, take the needed time to purposefully consider what was communicated and then respond thoughtfully.

- *Unveil the Unknown*: You have your areas of experience and expertise that create your personal context. Stay mindful that your audience often has different experiences and expertise, so when you need to communicate something outside of the audience's experience or expertise base, get in their head by creating a story, an analogy or an example that meets them where they are and then make the point you were trying to make.

- *Value the Visual*: If 55 per cent of the impact in communication is non-verbal[*], you should also pay attention with your eyes, not just your ears and mouth, right? If there is a gap between the words and body language, trust what the body language is telling you.
- *Weigh Your Words*: Having just said that body language trumps the words, still, words obviously matter. Keep them simple and constructive.
- *X-Ray Exceptions*: Stay focussed on the bigger picture. Do not allow the rare exceptions to dominate the communication.
- *Yield the You*: Communication essentially implies there are at least two people in the mix. What if you looked at things from the other person's point of view? What if you told the person what you were thinking about or what your intentions were? It would mean you put the other person before you. Essentially, you yield. And once you do, you will discover you will also get 'yielded to'.

---

[*]Ashenden, Pauline, 'Nonverbal Communication: How Body Language & Nonverbal Cues Are Key', *lifesize*, 18 February 2020, http://tinyurl.com/59ure8tk. Accessed on 6 February 2024.

- *Zoom to Zero*: You can master the A–Zs of constructive communication. But we are human. And an important part of being human is making mistakes. But mistakes do not mean that we cannot backtrack! We can always turn around and start over. Or do over. Go back to the beginning. Let bygones be bygones. You will be in a much better place. So…ready to start? There is no time like the present.

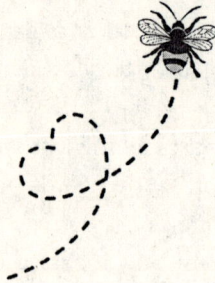

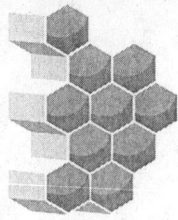

Bee Attitude #7

Bee Curious

Ask questions about your job and the organization respectfully. Seek out information and resources that will help you reach your full potential.

Follow the action items given below diligently to follow through on this Bee Attitude:

- When starting a new role, remember curiosity is a great path to learning.
- Many people think questions show weakness, but in truth, questions show engagement, quest for learning, interest in the topic and a willingness to try.
- Someone who asks natural questions will be viewed more positively than someone who just listens and observes.
- Focus on learning the work. When you are on a quest to learn, it will make you less distracted.
- Strive to learn from others. Determine what they do that you want to mimic and what you want to avoid.
- Ask about best practices from those who have recently travelled through the path you are on. Ask them about challenges and lessons learnt.
- Inquire about advice others would have if they were starting over.

- Remember, questions are viewed by organizations as an essential part of the learning journey.
- Create a new habit of asking questions every day.
- Listen with the intention of learning.
- Be known as the curious one.
- Remember, if you ask the questions, you must listen and retain the answers as well.
- People can get frustrated when the same questions are asked over and over and the receiver does not learn from the questions. Note the repetition of your questions.
- Take notes to help you remember the answers. Review your notes on a regular basis.
- Offer to teach others who follow in your footsteps to anchor your learning.
- Use curiosity as a starting point for building relationships.
- Curiosity in the spirit of learning is a great skill for both the learner and the team.
- Someone who models a genuine, curious spirit is often viewed as inviting, engaged and committed to learning.
- Be curious when you meet someone new. Instead of talking about yourself, activate your curious nature and learn about the other person.
- In moments of curiosity, listen to learn and discover the uniqueness of the other person.
- Utilize curiosity with new co-workers and even your manager. Break out of the ritual patterns of the check-in dialogue and turn on your curiosity mindset.
- Surprise your colleagues and activate curiosity with

genuine interest. Ask follow-up questions you may have seldom asked earlier. Dig a little deeper into the responses.

- Be aware of missed opportunities of expressing curiosity. These are those moments when someone makes a statement, and instead of following up with a genuine question the listener just lets it fade away.

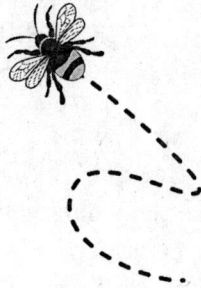

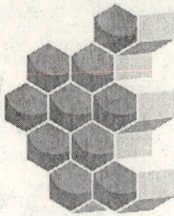

Bee Attitude #8

Bee Frank

Balance honesty with a spirit of being considerate. Follow the action items given below diligently to follow through on this Bee Attitude:

- When people are new to a role or job, they tend to default to being quiet rather than speaking up in meetings. Practise finding your voice and offer an opinion during discussions. Set a goal to increase your meeting participation before each meeting.
- In a work setting, be honest with your leader. Don't assume that they know what is wrong with you or how you are feeling. Your leader is not a mind reader. Let them know what is working for you and where you may be challenged. Establish an honesty baseline with your manager.
- Plan your thoughts in advance. Preparation will help you create a clear and compassionate message.
- Consider the best way to use candour with your peers and boss. The delivery of your message may need to be adjusted based on how you feel it will be received.
- Avoid hinting as a means of feedback. Many people tend to talk in circles and hope the receiver is picking up the subtle hints.

- Use a feedback loop to check for understanding, to be certain your message was delivered and that the intent of the message was received. You can say something along the lines of: 'Based on what I just said, please share what you understood and how that feels for you.'

- Be honest with co-workers and friends. In organizations, it can sometimes be challenging to find someone who will be completely honest with no agenda except to help. Be the person people can go to for unfiltered feedback. Be honest and compassionate with the intent to help someone gain awareness and insight.

- Don't ramble. Keep your thoughts clear and concise. Spend your words wisely.

- When being frank, pick one topic to speak clearly on at a time.

- Speak your truth with respect and kindness.

- Ask the person you are talking to if they are open to an observation. Recognize whether this person might appreciate hearing feedback that could be of value to one's success. If unsure, ask if they would be open to feedback that may be helpful.

- Discover your blind spots. Ask for feedback from others. Allow someone you respect to provide a few behaviours that would help you become more successful. Sometimes, we are not aware of our own roadblocks.

- Own your feedback. If you think it and share it, then own it. Don't blame the feedback you give on others.

- Don't speak for the collective group. Even if you

know that others may share your viewpoint, only speak from your experience.

- Provide feedback in the spirit of helpfulness. When coming from a place of genuine helpfulness, people tend to receive the message more positively.

- Practise your message. If you have a difficult message for someone, practise how you will share this message.

- Keep the message specific and concise. Be aware of your reaction to the 'awkwardness' of the conversation. Don't over-communicate or rationalize the issue.

- If someone is frank and honest with you, thank them for their willingness to share their comments with you. We can't learn and grow if we don't know.

- Listen to how you respond to feedback from others. Do you find yourself defending your words and behaviours, or trying to validate and prove yourself right? You don't always have to agree with the feedback, but a great question to ask yourself is, 'What can I learn here?'

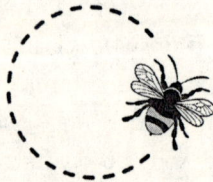

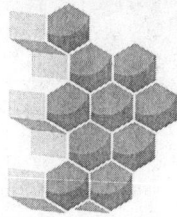

Bee Attitude #9

Bee Kind

Seek to uplift others. Maintain a spirit of gentleness. Give the benefit of the doubt. Give smiles. Say thank you and please. Give your time to someone. Truly listen. Follow the action items given below diligently to follow through on this Bee Attitude:

- When people meet you for the first time, remember that they are forming an impression of you at the very beginning of your relationship.
- Personal awareness of what kindness looks like, sounds like and feels like is the beginning of making a difference for those in your personal circle. Evaluate what kindness looks like to you and how you demonstrate it every day. Then you can determine what you want to start, stop and continue doing.
- Be yourself and make sure your kindness shows in your facial expressions too. There is no extra charge for a smile that reaches the eyes. Body language is a major component of communication.
- Remember that kindness is the personal culture you create with others. It is the spirit of giving, helpfulness and genuine caring that you exhibit day in and out.
- Kindness consistency matters! Be careful not to derail

your kindness culture with a bad day or an emotional outburst on the regular.

- Gain clarity of your values and how you want people to see you. List the behaviours you need to be demonstrating daily to create your kindness legacy.
- Kindness during good times is easy. Pay extra attention to how you respond when frustrated or under pressure.
- Think about the impact you want to have on those around you and how a kindness role model impacts an organization.
- Give your kindness away! Make a commitment to demonstrate kindness at least five times each day. Then, watch the ripple effect like a pebble in a pond.
- Your behaviours are your choice. Whether positive or negative, you choose the behaviour you want to activate. What will you choose?
- Talk with a trusted friend and share that you are working on creating your own kindness culture. Ask for feedback when this person witnesses your kindness in action.

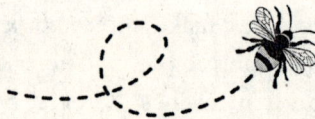

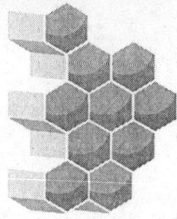

Bee Attitude #10

Bee Humble

Maintain personal pride in your work without boasting. Give credit to others and put others first when you can.

Follow the action items given below diligently to follow through on this Bee Attitude:

- Identify your strengths. Know how you can add value and contribute to the team.
- Recognize the value in the adage 'many hands make light work'.
- Invite others in and celebrate everyone's differences.
- Remember that very seldom do we accomplish success just by ourselves.
- Think about the people who have opened doors for you and been your advocate.
- Remember those who saw something special in you before you recognized it in yourself.
- Consider who had a positive influence on your life and helped you get where you are today. Make sure to thank them.
- Look around you and find where you can offer your support and assistance.
- Listen openly without an agenda. This will help you

discover where you can offer the most assistance.

- Live with a willingness to help from behind the scenes.
- Find ways to offer your strengths and spotlight the strengths of others.
- Point out the many attributes that contributed to team success.
- Be open to new ideas.
- Recognize that you don't have all the answers and be willing to learn.
- Catch yourself in those moments when you seek the limelight, praise or adoration of others.
- Stay in alignment with your values, priorities and ultimate goals.
- Be mindful of your lucky breaks and find ways to give back to others.
- Remember those moments when you had to work extremely hard and push past incredible challenges. In those moments, you were a humble warrior.
- Stay aware of the situations that trigger a more self-focussed mindset.
- Ask yourself: 'What is an accomplishment for me?'
- Never take credit for a project that involved many people.
- Have you ever felt that you do not receive enough positive feedback, so you feel the need to elaborate on your value? If so, consider the impression this has on others.
- Beware of boasting and singing your own praises. Do you hunger for the accolades of others? If so, ask yourself why.
- Identify how you can find value in your work, without

needing the praise of others. (For example: accomplished projects, growth of others, celebration events)

- Be sure to stay humble and don't overuse your strengths in a way that could be interpreted as arrogant or self-serving.
- Recognize that there will always be someone with more experience, knowledge and expertise in the room. Also remember that that is okay.

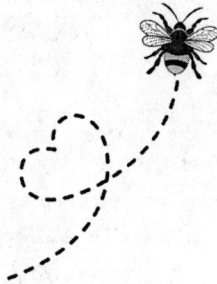

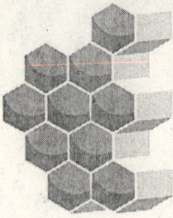

Bee Attitude #11

Bee Ambitious

Without violating the principles listed in 'Bee Humble', compete to be your best self every day.

Follow the action items given below diligently to follow through on this Bee Attitude:

- As you begin your career, recognize that it is okay to want to progress through your career.
- It is important to be your own advocate. Don't depend on others to guide you through your career as this is **your journey**! It is your responsibility to learn and determine what is right for you.
- If you don't know what you want to do, start talking with those who seem to be a few steps further in their journey.
- Do your homework and learn about different positions within the organization.
- Discover your strengths and identify what things seem to fuel you.
- Ask yourself, 'What work activities am I drawn to?'
- Determine which jobs and activities pique your curiosity.
- Recognize that failures get you closer to your goal. It is part of the growing process.

- Be proactive and converse with a senior employee about their journey.
- Ask for advice and best practices that they might recommend.
- Say YES to take on a new project even if you feel unprepared. One caveat here is to make sure you balance additional responsibilities against potential burnout.
- Volunteer to help others so you can learn.
- Bring a learning mindset to all jobs.
- Recognize that mistakes are part of the learning journey. Don't let them get you down.
- Learn from your mistakes and celebrate progress.
- Challenge yourself to step out of your comfort zone.
- Treat others with respect and kindness as you move through your career.
- Never show disrespect or speak in a critical or condescending manner.
- Evaluate your skills to determine where your strengths and opportunities are.
- Be confident in telling others about your varied interests.
- Challenge yourself to strengthen your strengths even further. This is where momentum is created.
- Learn how to manage your weaknesses or challenge areas. You don't need to make your weaknesses your strengths, but you do need to develop a level of skill to avoid roadblocks.

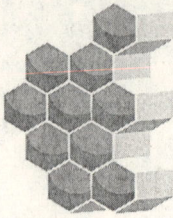

Bee Attitude #12

Bee a Team Player

Think of any team sport. It takes every individual at every position to do their job for the team to succeed. Know your role and others' roles as well. When another player is down, pick them up. Integrate your strengths into the work. Allow others to assist you with any weaknesses.

Follow the action items given below diligently to follow through on this Bee Attitude:

- Remember the value of 'We Bee' versus 'Me Bee'.
- Describe your contribution to the team. Determine if you are helpful, supportive, invisible or a distraction.
- List the positive attributes you bring to your team.
- Behave well in meetings. That can mean different things in different organizations. Watch and learn.
- If you are not speaking up now, what are you waiting for? What needs to happen for you to bring your 'team-player' spirit?
- A team player wears many hats. There are times to talk, to listen, to ask questions, to observe, to speak up and to share a different viewpoint. What do you typically do?
- How would you describe the energy you bring to a

team? Does it show up in more of a positive way, a neutral way or a negative way?

- Don't be critical of others. Share opinions with others on your team in a positive tone.
- What kind of influence do you have as a team member?
- Determine how you want to be viewed by your team and take action.

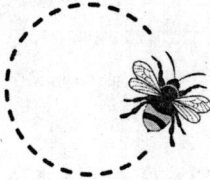

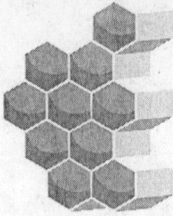

Bee Attitude #13

Bee Independent

Without violating the principles described in 'Bee a Team player', be self-aware and self-motivated, so as to remain independent.

Follow the action items given below diligently to follow through on this Bee Attitude:

- While teamwork is important, there may be times when you need to work independently and take care of matters on your own.
- Sometimes, the team and organization need you to bring your best work, so others can pick up where you leave off.
- When you embrace your gifts or strengths, it ignites your internal motivation to work independently and get things accomplished.
- Recognize the importance of good decisions. When you are aware of your skills, this increases your self-confidence which is the catalyst for better decision-making.
- Evaluate the level of confidence you have in your work. Assess how you can raise that level of confidence.
- Count on self-motivation for doing outstanding work.

- On a scale of 1 (Low) to 10 (high), rate your confidence to work independently. If your answer is a 7 or less, consider asking your supervisor for some pointers.
- Create a mechanism to monitor your output and keep track of expectations.

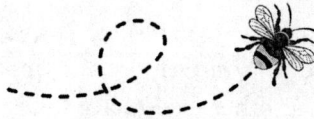

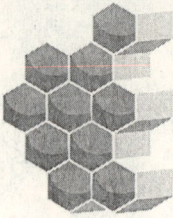

Bee Attitude #14

Bee Enthusiastic

Bring good energy to your work consistently. Communicate positively consistently. Recognize and respect that other bees have different perspectives. Inspire other bees and celebrate their successes.

Follow the action items given below diligently to follow through on this Bee Attitude:

- As a new hire, pay attention to your enthusiasm level.
- Accept the tasks you are given with a smile and a readiness to learn.
- Think about how enthusiasm shows up for you and what others see, hear and feel from you.
- Listen to your dialogue and how you speak with others. Do you bring energy to a discussion (as the enthusiastic team member), provide no energy at all (as the silent observer) or do you drain energy from the group with your words and behaviours (as the 'this won't work' team member)?
- Enthusiasm comes from deep within and it looks different on everyone, depending on one's natural style. Both introverts and extroverts can be enthusiastic.
- For some people, enthusiasm is more visible and outwardly focussed and can easily be observed due

to one's tone of voice, volume, facial expressions, physical gestures and overall energy.

- Others may be enthusiastic as well, but it may show up differently based on what is comfortable for their natural style. In this instance, enthusiasm may be more internally driven, like increased energy towards the task at hand, purposeful learning, increased level of engagement, dedicated attention to detail or a drive for specific results.

- For some, enthusiasm may be observed through their dedicated service to others. You may notice that these individuals are extremely driven to helping, volunteering, caring for and quietly making a difference for others behind the scenes. Enthusiasm and compassion in action is seen through these individuals.

- In the work setting, enthusiasm has many faces as well. It is mostly viewed as a positive attribute.

- Awareness is critical. Enthusiasm is important, but for those who display the outward signs of enthusiasm (the extrovert group), they may want to be aware of their co-workers' styles and not 'overdo' the enthusiasm metre. Too much of a good thing can become a distraction.

- Someone who is enthusiastic at work may be identified as someone who approaches work with an attitude of joy.

- Optimism and enthusiasm tend to be at the same party.

- Warning: Enthusiasm can be contagious to those in close proximity.

- Keep in mind, people choose how they approach their work. Those who approach work with an enthusiastic spirit tend to draw people in and bring an increased level of joy to the workplace.
- Enthusiasm is helpful for team cohesion as well. During heavy workload times, enthusiasm can help lift the emotional burden and provide inspiration and momentum to get the work accomplished.

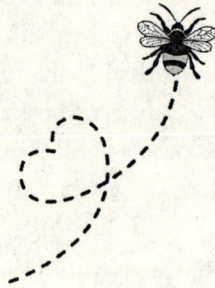

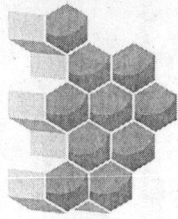

Bee Attitude #15

Bee Committed

Review the Bee Attitudes above and then look in the mirror.

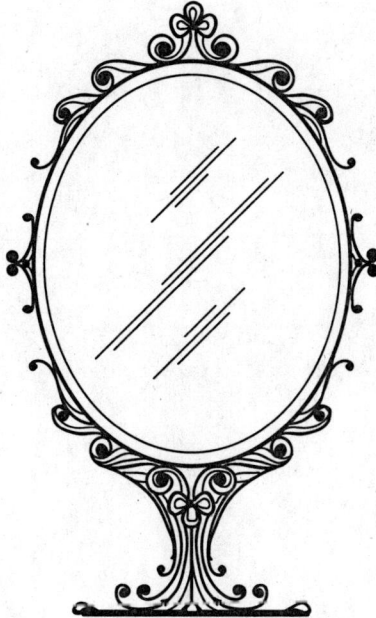

SELF-PERCEPTION RATING

Now that we have the common working definitions, rate yourself on a scale of 1 (Poor) to 10 (Excellent) in each Bee Attitude:

	(Poor)									(Excellent)
Beeing Knowledgeable	1	2	3	4	5	6	7	8	9	10
Beeing Dependable	1	2	3	4	5	6	7	8	9	10
Beeing Flexible	1	2	3	4	5	6	7	8	9	10
Beeing Innovative	1	2	3	4	5	6	7	8	9	10
Beeing Authentic	1	2	3	4	5	6	7	8	9	10
Beeing a Great Communicator	1	2	3	4	5	6	7	8	9	10
Beeing Curious	1	2	3	4	5	6	7	8	9	10
Beeing Frank	1	2	3	4	5	6	7	8	9	10
Beeing Kind	1	2	3	4	5	6	7	8	9	10
Beeing Humble	1	2	3	4	5	6	7	8	9	10
Beeing Ambitious	1	2	3	4	5	6	7	8	9	10
Beeing a Team Player	1	2	3	4	5	6	7	8	9	10
Beeing Independent	1	2	3	4	5	6	7	8	9	10
Beeing Enthusiastic	1	2	3	4	5	6	7	8	9	10
Beeing Committed	1	2	3	4	5	6	7	8	9	10

If you rated yourself a 7 or less in any category, it is time to get the mirror out and take a deeper look. Go to the corresponding 'Bee Attitude' and look for ideas to improve in the respective category.

CROSS RATINGS

This is often a harder test compared to the previous one. The test itself is not more difficult but digesting the results might be. In your team or your department, make copies of the survey and set it up so that one or more persons anonymously rates you on a scale of 1 (Poor) to 10 (Excellent) in each Bee Attitude. Maintaining the anonymity of the ratings is important!

	(Poor)									(Excellent)
Beeing Knowledgeable	1	2	3	4	5	6	7	8	9	10
Beeing Dependable	1	2	3	4	5	6	7	8	9	10
Beeing Flexible	1	2	3	4	5	6	7	8	9	10
Beeing Innovative	1	2	3	4	5	6	7	8	9	10
Beeing Authentic	1	2	3	4	5	6	7	8	9	10
Beeing a Great Communicator	1	2	3	4	5	6	7	8	9	10
Beeing Curious	1	2	3	4	5	6	7	8	9	10
Beeing Frank	1	2	3	4	5	6	7	8	9	10
Beeing Kind	1	2	3	4	5	6	7	8	9	10

Beeing Humble	1		2	3	4	5	6	7	8	9		10
Beeing Ambitious	1		2	3	4	5	6	7	8	9		10
Beeing a Team Player	1		2	3	4	5	6	7	8	9		10
Beeing Independent	1		2	3	4	5	6	7	8	9		10
Beeing Enthusiastic	1		2	3	4	5	6	7	8	9		10
Beeing Committed	1		2	3	4	5	6	7	8	9		10

If you were rated a 7 or less in any category, it is time to get the mirror out and take a deeper look. Go to the corresponding 'Bee Attitude' and look for ideas to improve in the respective category.

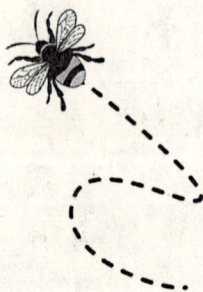